Aging Together

Dementia, Friendship, and Flourishing Communities

Susan H. McFadden

and

John T. McFadden

Johns Hopkins University Press

Baltimore

Johns Hopkins Paperback edition, 2014
2 4 6 8 9 7 5 3 1

All scriptural quotations are taken from the New Revised
Standard Version Bible.

Johns Hopkins University Press
2715 North Charles Street
Baltimore, Maryland 21218-4363
www.press.jhu.edu

The Library of Congress has cataloged the hardcover edition of this book as follows:
McFadden, Susan H., author.
Aging together : dementia, friendship, and flourishing communities /
Susan H. McFadden and John T. McFadden.
p. ; cm.
Includes bibliographical references and index.
ISBN-13: 978-0-8018-9986-7 (hardcover : alk. paper)
ISBN-10: 0-8018-9986-9 (hardcover : alk. paper)
1. Dementia—Patients—Family relationships.   2. Dementia—Social
aspects.   I. McFadden, John T., author.   II. Title.
[DNLM: 1. Alzheimer Disease—therapy.   2. Aged—psychology.
3. Alzheimer Disease—psychology.   4. Community Networks.   5. Social
Support.   6. Spirituality. WT 155]
RC521.M44 2011
362.196'83—dc22   2010045133

A catalog record for this book is available from the British Library.

ISBN-13: 978-1-4214-1375-4
ISBN-10: 1-4214-1375-2

Special discounts are available for bulk purchases of this book. For more information,
please contact Special Sales at 410-516-6936 or specialsales@press.jhu.edu.

Johns Hopkins University Press uses environmentally friendly book materials,
including recycled text paper that is composed of at least 30 percent
post-consumer waste, whenever possible.

CONTENTS

We were married in January 1970, halfway through our senior year in college. It was the era of the Vietnam War, utopian back-to-the-land dreams, and "sex, drugs, and rock-and-roll." Ours was a cohort not much given to career planning or long-term goals. The shadow cast by the war and our collective certainty that the Age of Aquarius was dawning made us prone to heed Baba Ram Dass's admonition to "Be here now."

As is often true for college cohorts, our anchor in the sea of chaos swirling about us was our community of friends, in our case a motley crew of hippies, political activists, musicians, intellectuals, and goat farmers who collectively constituted our "tribe." And like many other generations of college students, we held the conceit that we were unique and that the special bonds we shared would bind us to one another for all of our lives. We joked that one day we would all reside together in the "rock-and-roll nursing home," where we would sit in rocking chairs on the front porch and argue about which album to play next. "No more Beatles! Put on some Hendrix!" Such lines were delivered in our best approximations of an aged voice, with one hand cupped behind an ear and the other bracing "the bum knee where the rheumitiz is actin' up again."

It was a lighthearted fantasy designed to sustain courage and hope. Somehow we would make it through those frightening times, drawing strength from one another, before ultimately reuniting as a community to share our collective vision of the good life. But our fantasies of the rock-and-roll nursing home never took into account the possibility of dementia. Our imaginations could extend only to diminished hearing, wrinkled skin, and creaky joints. Aging would take some toll on our bodies, but we never entertained the possibility that we might not remain the same "selves" we were at age twenty.

Those friends from 1970 are now widely scattered. Some are retired from successful careers, while a few never strayed far from the goat farm. Several have died. We are in regular contact with only a handful as we now move further into our sixties. Who among this once-inseparable community will be the first to be diagnosed with dementia?

By grace or good fortune, we found our own way into adulthood. John attended theological school and was ordained a minister in the United Church of Christ, serving large congregations in New Jersey and Wisconsin for a total of thirty-four years. Susan earned an M.A. in experimental psychology and a Ph.D. in psychology and religion before entering academic life with a particular focus on adult development and aging. Our two children are now well into adulthood themselves, and one recently gave birth to our first grandchild.

With much of our life together centered in congregations, we have been privileged to spend far more time in the company of older adults than most members of our cohort. When we were impoverished students, older adults of the congregation reached out to us in friendship, inviting us for meals and gifting us with used clothing. When we moved into our first parsonage, it was the "old ladies" of the congregation who filled it with furniture. As unpolished young "flower children," we were grateful to be invited to elegant parties hosted by persons in their seventies, who schooled us in the social graces. We have been richly blessed in countless ways by participating in intergenerational communities all of our adult lives.

As we enter the "third age" of our shared life (the period of life bounded at one end by retirement from primary occupation and at the other by decline in physical or cognitive health), we find ourselves delighting in new friendships with persons younger than we are. Too often friendships between different age cohorts are reduced to clichés of one-way relationships, either positively (elder as dispenser of wisdom and guidance) or negatively (elder as care receiver). Wisdom and care are both given and received in all relationships, and friendships across the lines of generation offer special riches. Further, these friendships are best nurtured and supported in the embrace of flourishing communities of persons who honestly acknowledge their vulnerabilities and love one another nevertheless.

Our aim in this book is to present a radical view of friendship that is not based on obvious reciprocity or shared memories. We usually assume that one of the most important components of a friendship is that another person has known us through time. Friends help us to know who we are; they represent a part of our selfhood. However, when considering relationships with persons who have dementia, we are forced to ask how it is possible to be a friend with someone who does not remember us from moment to moment, even though together we may have spun a web of friendship over many years. Can we still be friends? And, can we make new friends with persons at various points in the dementia process, persons who may not be able to put together a story about how we met, what we have done together, and why we are important to each other? Can any meaning be gained from cultivating such friendships?

These questions will become more pressing in the coming years as the greatest number of persons in human history enters old age. Unfortunately, we live in a time when we separate persons from one another in later life—psychologically, socially, and physically—by using criteria based on brain health. It is not hard to tally up the positive ways friends who age successfully enrich our lives. But, is it possible that friendship with persons who have dementia—either those we have known a long time or persons newly met—might add meaning to the experience of aging? The answer is yes, and this book aims to show how this kind of friendship is possible.

We begin with an introductory chapter that offers more detail about what we call our "standing grounds" in academic psychology and pastoral theology. These provide the perspectives we employ in examining the challenges the future will present to people who call one another "friend." After offering a cursory review of various types of dementia diagnoses in Chapter 1 (a kind of "Dementia 101," which we realize will quickly become outdated, given the rapid accumulation of research and clinical observations), in Chapter 2 we consider what it feels like to receive the diagnosis.

Throughout the chapters we illustrate our points with stories about people we have known. Of course, we use no actual names, but we hope these small vignettes give a taste of what some call the "lived experience" of dementia.

We begin to answer yes to our question about the possibility of retaining friendship in the face of memory loss when we examine the reasons we value human beings, in Chapter 3. If others are valuable to us only because they possess a part of our individual genetic code or because they can reciprocate our altruism, then there is little reason for friendship with persons who have dementia. This friendship *is* possible, however, if it is infused with the belief that persons should be valued regardless of their intellectual status and that personhood itself is grounded in relationship.

Chapter 4 takes us into a detailed discussion of friendship from two very different points of view: contemporary social scientific research and Aristotle's reflections on friendship in the *Nicomachean Ethics*. We continue with those two perspectives in Chapter 5 as we look more deeply into the challenges raised when a friend experiences memory loss and confusion.

We do not want to be facile in our encouragement of friendship, and thus in Chapter 6, we acknowledge the fear and anxiety evoked by thinking about dementia in ourselves and those we love. Chapter 6 explores the psychological and cultural sources of these feelings and their effects on those who are living with dementia. Chapter 7 moves us beyond fear and anxiety by showing how these feelings that distance us from friends can be transformed into love and compassion for our friends.

Chapter 8 begins to push the discussion in a new direction by examining the contours of communities that can best support people through the trials and tests of late-life friendship, especially when dementia is introduced into the picture. We present a vision of the flourishing community, one that centers on the practices of hospitality and the acceptance of all persons regardless of physical or mental status. In Chapter 9, we show that religious congregations might be models of flourishing communities, although we realize that, like any human institution, they too can become afflicted with petty and not-so-petty conflict. Nevertheless, we see possibilities for congregations to show the wider community a new vision of friendship with persons who are living with dementia. The world's faith traditions teach that humans have value that transcends material existence and that remains in even the most debilitated individual. Under these conditions, meaning and human value are not mere abstract philosophical or religious constructions, but rather they infuse the space between one human being seeking love and another freely offering it.

We need to be clear from the outset that this book is written by two people who are Christian, a statement we hope can be read in the United States without association with narrow-minded, true-believer culture warriors. Throughout the book, we discuss emerging theological scholarship about how disability can be reconstructed within a religious worldview. At the same time, we realize that religious organizations are both inclusive and exclusive when it comes to persons who are "different," whether because of physical or mental disability or other categories of identity that often separate persons from one another. In plain language, congregations can be mean and religious people can be hateful. This applies to all religious traditions. We are not uncritical about our particular faith tradition, but we will show how certain contemporary Christian theologians have made important contributions to our thinking about dementia, friendship, and community. At the same time, we acknowledge that we have much to learn from other religious perspectives. For example, Rabbi Dayle Friedman's writings (2001a, 2005, 2008) about Jewish pastoral care have strongly influenced our thinking about the personhood of those who have dementia.

Friedman uses the Hebrew term *livui ruchani* to describe pastoral care as spiritual accompaniment. This way of being present to others is not confined to ministers and rabbis—the persons we usually think of as "pastors." Rather, she explains that *luv* as used in biblical and rabbinical texts refers to those who walk with others. These can include "ministering angels, God's presence, friends, priests, and peers" (2005, xvii). This idea of accompaniment works well with the metaphor we are using in this book—the dementia road. People who have received a diagnosis of dementia need others to make this journey with them. However, given the implied reciprocity of friendship, we also need a vision of how people who are experiencing the challenges of dementia can offer spiritual accompaniment to those who have few memory difficulties. In other words, we can help one another along this road together.

Although we are focusing on aging and dementia in this book, in actuality, people travel many kinds of difficult roads with their friends. Some wind through the territory of terrible losses, mental illness, cancer, divorce, and myriad other ways humans suffer. They listen as friends pour out their sorrow, fear, regret, guilt, anger. They visit friends in hospitals, prisons, and homes. They enter friends' names in scheduling programs and make phone calls, write notes, send emails. They connect with them through MySpace, Facebook, and specialized networking/support sites like CaringBridge. In other words, in no way do we mean to imply that people are not already accompanying friends through challenging terrains, although there are many cases in which people feel abandoned in their despair by persons whom they once called friends but who turn away when troubles mount. Moreover, we are not trying to rank suffering, saying one form is worse than another. Instead, we are addressing a condition that some researchers and clinicians believe will be diagnosed with increasing frequency as the largest cohort in history ages.

The speed of change in the twenty-first century threatens to leave older persons behind, especially those who have memory loss. That is why it is necessary to think about the things that abide, and we take up that topic in Chapter 10. These things are faith, hope, and love, and we situate them within a world in which increasing numbers of persons are receiving the diagnosis of some form of dementia at increasingly earlier ages.

Although this is not a "how to" book, Chapter 11 offers a number of concrete suggestions about remaining in friendship with those diagnosed with dementia as well as with their family members, who themselves can sometimes react negatively to what friends perceive as well-intentioned advice or offers of help. In addition, the chapter suggests the possibility of making new friends with persons who are living with this chronic affliction, and it shows how friends can contribute to the formation of flourishing communities.

We hope by the time readers reach the end of this book that they will clearly understand our position: that it is possible, necessary, and rewarding to have meaningful relationships with persons who are traveling the dementia road. The last chapter examines how forgetting can be a blessing and how both memory and forgetting require us to consider our experience of time itself. We compare two models of time—*chronos* time and *kairos* time—and discuss how we might negotiate the tension between them in our relationships with friends who have dementia. Dementia does not have to be seen as an individual tragedy. Instead, it can be understood as an experience of personal change that occurs within community. If communities are to flourish, then they must extend hospitality to all, including persons who struggle with memory loss. Their lives have worth and value, and they have much to teach their friends about love.

ACKNOWLEDGMENTS

The idea of coauthoring a book that would bring together our respective disciplines (the psychology of aging; theology and pastoral care) was decades in gestation. We believed that each had rich resources to offer to a much-needed conversation about how we can age together as friends within flourishing communities, especially given that dementia will inevitably be a component of our shared journey of aging. Our hope was that together we might offer a broad perspective that drew from the riches of philosophy, the insights of psychology and other social sciences, and the wisdom of the world's faith traditions. Our fear was that we might produce a manuscript that was neither fish nor fowl—too academic for the general reader and too broad for an academic audience. If we have succeeded in finding an appropriate balance, it is because we have received a great deal of help from our friends along the way.

This is a book about friendship, and we have been blessed with many friends. Some we have cherished for many decades, and some we have come to know only in recent years. We have had friends older than our parents, many of whom have now passed from this life, and some of our friends are younger than our children.

We are especially grateful to our friends who have already made significant contributions to this new conversation about aging and dementia. Anne Basting, Dayle Friedman, and Elizabeth MacKinlay have been our teachers and sources of inspiration. Another teacher-friend is geriatric psychiatrist Abhilash Desai, who offers gifts of hope and even joy to the many persons he diagnoses as having dementia. We thank the staff of the Alzheimer's Center of Excellence in Appleton, Wisconsin, for carrying on his important work. We also thank the residents and staff of Evergreen Retirement Community in Oshkosh, Wisconsin, and Brewster Village in Appleton, Wisconsin, for sharing their stories and offering us hospitality and support.

Susan extends appreciation to all the people who graciously agreed to be interviewed during her sabbatical and whose stories enrich this work. In addition, this book could not have been completed without the help of several persons at the University of Wisconsin, Oshkosh: Mary Bleser, Academic Department Associate of the Psychology Department; graduate assistant Ben Mullins, who retrieved articles and checked references; and the library staff, especially those who manage interlibrary loans. Several friends graciously offered to read early versions of chapters and provided helpful feedback: Joan Jensen, Helen McKean, and Lorain Giles.

John offers special thanks to Stanley Hauerwas, who inspired him to think theologically about dementia and served as a sounding board for ideas he was exploring. He received encouragement from many other friends in the Ekklesia Project, including Kyle Childress, Joel Shuman, and Brian Volck. He is also grateful to Jeff Marks, of Brewster Village, who introduced him to the joy of sharing friendships with persons who are living with advanced dementia.

In addition to being a book about friendship, this work is about community. We have developed deep, meaningful connections with a variety of communities in which many friendships have been nurtured: the university, various professional aging organizations, and clergy groups. We are thankful for the congregations in which we were schooled in living "subversive" intergenerational friendships, especially First Congregational United Church of Christ in Appleton.

We also extend our appreciation to our editor, Wendy Harris, for believing in the value of this project and shepherding it along the way. She provided encouragement and support even before we had a glimmer of how this undertaking would unfold. Barbara Lamb, our copy editor, asked the right questions while making our manuscript tighter and cleaner, and perhaps finally taught us the distinction between *that* and *which*.

Finally, we are grateful for a road: Route 29, the long and boring highway that extends from our home in eastern Wisconsin to Minnesota, where our children live. Often in the course of this tedious drive we found time to talk about the themes we explore in this book (occasionally missing our exit when the conversation became passionate). We suspect that several of our images—traveling the dementia road, for example—owe their genesis in part to Route 29.

Aging Together

Introduction

"I've got a story for you!" This was the opening greeting from a woman calling to talk about an upsetting recent experience that involved her husband, who has lived with the diagnosis of Alzheimer's disease for about three years. She knew that we were writing a book about friendship and community and she had met one of us at an Alzheimer's Association meeting several months earlier. Her story unfolded quickly as she described how much her husband loved to bowl. Seeking some kind of activity they could enjoy together and that would provide exercise, she had signed up for a mixed bowling league. Her husband was skilled at bowling, even though he occasionally had to be reminded that it was his turn. Nevertheless, she reported, "he helps us win." However, the manager of the bowling alley had just telephoned to say that one of the women in the league—a person she had known for years in her church and thought of as a friend—had asked to bowl on another team, with people who were "normal." What was even more distressing was that the woman who wanted to switch leagues said that people like her husband "even forget they are married."

Our caller was justifiably hurt and angry. She considered calling her priest to talk about this behavior by a fellow church member, but she said, "he'd deny it." She wanted us to know that "the message isn't getting through" in the local community about how persons can continue to enjoy life and remain in friendship despite having memory loss and confusion.

We have heard many tales like this. The stories can be heartrending, the terms are confusing, the numbers are dizzying, and the topic elicits so much anxiety that some people say they would rather think about death. We are talking about *dementia*, a general term signifying progressive forgetfulness and the confusion that attends forgetfulness. Although various medical conditions can cause forgetfulness and confusion at any age, today the word *dementia* is generally associated with older adults' loss of memory and other related cognitive functions.[1]

Alzheimer's disease is the most commonly diagnosed form of dementia, having first been described at the beginning of the twentieth century. However, until the mid-twentieth century, people spoke of "senility" or "senile dementia" when describing the behavior of an elderly person who could not recall recent events, follow a conversation, or maintain regular daily activities and who in general showed a loss of vitality.[2] Adding to this confusing mix of labels, late in the nineteenth century psychiatrists began to use the term *dementia praecox,* or *premature dementia,* when referring to persons who today would probably receive the diagnosis of schizophrenia. Currently, those rare persons who exhibit symptoms of memory loss in middle adulthood may be diagnosed as having young-onset Alzheimer's disease, which is a kind of inherited premature dementia, although it bears no resemblance to the way we currently conceive of schizophrenia.[3] Finally, to add one more element of confusion to this picture, in the late twentieth century a new category describing memory problems associated with aging emerged: *amnestic mild cognitive impairment* (MCI). This describes a condition in which people complain of memory difficulties but function normally in their daily lives, even though they may score lower on memory tests than others their age who have no memory complaints (Petersen 2004).

In 2008, the Website of the National Institute on Aging (NIA) estimated that between 2.4 and 4.5 million Americans have Alzheimer's disease. In the same year, the Alzheimer's Association published its "facts and figures" report online and raised the estimate of Americans who have Alzheimer's to 5.2 million. The cover page of the report proclaims that 10 million baby boomers will develop Alzheimer's, and inside the report one learns that the number could go to 14 million if all types of dementia are included. Alzheimer's Disease International, an umbrella group for Alzheimer's associations worldwide, claimed in 2008 that 30 million people live with dementia, a number this organization projects will rise to 100 million by 2050.[4]

One question that almost always arises in discussions of aging and dementia is "How old is old?" According to the National Institute of Mental Health, about 10 percent of all Americans 65 or older live with Alzheimer's disease, but that estimate increases to 50 percent of persons 85 or older. Cutting the age figures another way, in 2008, two nationally representative studies by Brenda Plassman and colleagues at Duke University received considerable media attention. One estimated that 13.9 percent of all persons 71 years or older currently have dementia, and the other estimated the prevalence of mild cognitive impairment at 22.2 percent of those 71 or older (Plassman et al. 2007, 2008). Combining the findings of these two studies, Rob Stein, writing in the *Washington Post* (2008), concluded that "more than one-third of people 71 and older have some diminished mental function."

As a progressive illness that no therapy can yet reverse or prevent, dementia's theft of memory, reason, and autonomy is terrifying, especially when one distills the "big numbers" down to local communities. Imagine, for example, the fifty-fifth reunion of the high school class of 1966 (the year we graduated) being held in 2021. If 100 people attend that reunion, the research by Plassman and colleagues predicts that at least a dozen of them will have dementia and another 20 or so will be heading toward dementia, having begun to show signs of memory troubles without experiencing any debility in daily functioning. These men and women will be in their early seventies. Many will still be working, while others will have retired from paid employment but be actively involved in meaningful volunteer activities in their communities.

In this book, we refer frequently to the "dementia road." We use this metaphor for several reasons. First, it reflects the simple graphs one often sees on Websites (e.g., the NIA) and in books about Alzheimer's disease and other dementias.[5] They show the life span from birth to death, with two lines: one continues to chart a fairly straight course until about age 80, when there is a slight downward slope, indicating the normal changes in memory expected with increasing age. The other line diverges from the "healthy aging" line around age 55. It takes a more precipitous downward pathway, beginning with the label of "mild cognitive impairment" and ending with a notation about loss of independent function and death. These two lines are meant to indicate pathways through the aging process that split somewhere in midlife and never meet up again.

That the condition of the brain alone allows some people to age well and condemns others to age miserably is a relatively new notion. Nevertheless, the metaphor of the journey to describe the human experience of the passage of time has deep roots in Western history. As portrayed by cultural historian Thomas Cole (1992), this journey was once envisioned as a spiritual pilgrimage toward "communal ideals of transcendence" (xxx), but starting in the late nineteenth century, the focus shifted to the achievement and maintenance of individual health. Those never gifted with physical or mental health or those who lost it along the way were seen to have failed the moral tests of adulthood and aging.

We use the metaphor of the "dementia road" because it captures an evocative image coursing through theological, philosophical, historical, and literary works: aging as a journey. We also use this metaphor to raise the question of who walks this road. Is life really a "lonesome valley," like the folksong says? Granted, "nobody else can walk it for you," but other people can walk it *with* you. How far do those lines diverge? Can aging persons continue to have meaningful friendships and maintain vital communities even though some experience the accumulations of forgetfulness and others do not?

These questions are not being widely posed today. Most empirical research on the social relationships of persons who have dementia is directed toward families and paid caregivers. Philosophers, theologians, and other humanities scholars seeking to understand the self and community in our time generally do not think about aging and dementia. However, given the projected increase in cases, along with the proliferation of smaller, more complex family systems, it is time to consider the challenges dementia poses to friendships and community connections that have often been nurtured over the course of many decades. Will social stigma and personal fear sever these relationships? Or will people find the courage to walk the dementia road with one another, perhaps discovering along the way a deeper sense of meaning and value in friendship and community? Thinking back to that telephone call we received, will people who are living with dementia be forced to bowl alone?[6] These are the focal questions of this book.

Categories of Aging

Most people know at least a few older persons who are remarkably vital, physically fit, and intellectually astute—the ones who fit within the "healthy aging" group and who will not have to worry about what gerontologists call "normal age-related memory loss" until sometime in their eighties. These individuals are often portrayed in the media as exemplars of old age. They may think, There but for fortune go you or I, when they become aware of persons their age or younger who have veered away from the healthy aging path, or they may be persuaded that they have been rewarded for their temperance and good taste or, perhaps, their "good genes." Nevertheless, the ordinary frustrations of forgetfulness experienced by persons of all ages can be amplified even for this group, leading them to wonder occasionally, Will it happen to me? or What if it happens to someone close to me?

For persons in the second category, memory difficulties are more than a momentary source of annoyance. Although these persons may be functioning well in their everyday lives, repeated incidents of forgetfulness elicit concern (either their own or that of a loved one) and motivate them to "get it checked out." If they go to a memory clinic, they might be given a battery of neuropsychological tests and receive the diagnosis of MCI. However, MCI is not an established diagnosis in the *Diagnostic and Statistical Manual of Mental Disorders* (4th ed.), which, through the authority of its publisher, the American Psychiatric Association, determines the diagnoses used by physicians, insurance companies, researchers, and others.

Some clinicians are not persuaded that MCI is an actual disease condition, and they refuse to attach that label to their patients. Instead, they often recommend follow-up testing if memory problems continue and if no other medical problems known to cause memory difficulties are identified.[7] If there has been no improvement since the original tests or if there has been measurable decline, then these clinicians may diagnose early-stage Alzheimer's disease or, more vaguely, "cognitive disorder not otherwise specified."

Regardless of the diagnostic name given to their condition, most people will leave their doctor's office with a prescription for a drug that promises to slow the progression of forgetfulness. If they are fortunate, they will also be given information about community resources for themselves and their loved ones, as well as advice on diet and exercise. The very fortunate ones will have time to talk with a clinician who urges them to remain involved in their communities, engage in meaningful volunteer activities, pursue spiritual development, and find joy in being creative. According to the way we view dementia today, the aging journey for these people has veered across the border into what some with the diagnosis call "dementia land."[8]

People who go to memory clinics do so because they have some awareness that their memory is not as sharp as it once was. However, a recent study suggests that clinicians can pluck older people off the street randomly, administer some simple memory tests, and find that they meet the criteria for MCI. In other words, an older person may have no subjective awareness of memory problems but still be heading into "dementia land," according to a study of more than three thousand people living in Iowa (Purser, Fillenbaum, and Wallace 2006). They might *think* they belong among those in the "healthy aging" group, but perhaps they have already taken the downward turn in terms of the NIA cartography.

The final category into which older persons are often placed lies deep in the territory of dementia land. These individuals have been definitively diagnosed as having Alzheimer's disease, vascular dementia, Lewy body dementia, frontotemporal dementia, Huntington's disease, or any of the other rarer diseases that are usually placed under the umbrella term *dementia*. Their worlds have been radically reorganized by physical, emotional, cognitive, and social changes associated with memory loss, changes that often necessitate a move into the home of a relative or into long-term care. Although we will show that their lives can remain full of joy, meaning, and purpose, these persons are often viewed as being "other." Because their very existence can be terrifying to people who think they live in the land of the well, they are often shunned.[9]

Most books about aging today address these three categories separately, and the books themselves are often physically separated from one another. For example, a few years ago in a well-known bookstore in Portland, Oregon, we discovered that the books on mild cognitive impairment, Alzheimer's disease, and other dementias were located in a section labeled "neurology." In other words, these were defined as medical conditions. Someone had determined that they did not belong in the "aging" section, where several shelves of books promised readers sure-fire ways to stay young and fit and gave advice on how to preserve mental functions by eating fish three times a week, drinking red wine, exercising, volunteering, keeping in touch with friends, and doing crossword puzzles. We had no trouble finding the "aging" section, but we had to ask where the books about dementia were located.

In this book, we insist that all of these persons are aging together. Although we may create challenges for bookstore employees trying to decide where to place this work, nevertheless it is time to rethink the categories of aging. We are *all* aging, regardless of the balance of brain proteins and the state of neural fitness. By splitting aging persons into specific categories and giving them diagnostic labels, our culture has reinforced the sense of otherness in those whose mental functioning puts them below the cut-score of acceptable neuropsychological well-being. This "othering" threatens the bonds of friendship and community. Before we can understand this threat, however, we need to think deeply about how we understand friendship and how we envision a good community for all persons in the twenty-first century.

The categories of aging are not cultural abstractions or merely convenient ways of shelving books. They were created in the twentieth century as anxiety grew about "the stability and coherence of selfhood in general" (Ballenger 2006, 10) and as cosmic and communal meanings of old age disappeared (Moody 1986). Moreover, the old were not immune to these cultural changes. For example, Margaret Morganroth Gullette (2010) shared a poignant story of accompanying her elderly mother to dinner at a residential care community. Gullette overheard a woman nearby loudly proclaim that a male resident would not want to sit next to her mother because of her forgetfulness. In other words, healthy middle-aged people who fancy living into old age with full cognitive capacity are not the only ones who try to protect their own self-esteem by excluding those who remind them that progressive memory loss becomes more common as people grow older.

Standing Grounds

Over the course of the next two decades, the baby-boom cohort will be inexorably transitioning into what has traditionally been labeled "old age." In the social sciences, a *cohort* refers to a group of people born around the same time; the baby-boom cohort is defined by demographers as people born between 1946 and 1964. However, because it includes such a broad range of ages, worldviews, and experiences, some demographers divide it into the leading-edge baby boom and the late baby boom. People born in 1964 essentially "missed the '60s" in terms of the world that those born in the late 1940s encountered as they emerged into adulthood. Assuming they survive into old age, these people will all be 65 or older by 2030. Ever since the emergence of gerontology as a focus of interdisciplinary study in the middle of the twentieth century, the year 2030 has been treated as a demographer's touchstone. It represents that once nearly unimaginable year when, in the United States, one out of every five persons will be age 65 or older. Now, of course, 2030 does not seem so far away.

When the baby-boom cohort entered adulthood in the twentieth century, much turmoil erupted in societies around the world as this great mass of young people rebelled against authorities ranging from mom and dad to national governments. More quiet, but just as profoundly disturbing to many persons, was a shift—one might even describe it as a kind of consciousness raising—occurring in many outposts of academia. Scholars began to critique the tacit assumptions of their disciplines. Sometimes gathered under the broad rubric of *postmodernism,* this work reflected the thinking of French critical theorists, feminists, Marxists, and others whose views on literature, art, philosophy, and social science threatened the old order, which had been built on the authority of certain scholars and epistemologies reigning in Western thought since the Enlightenment.[10]

One of the outcomes of this new approach to scholarship has been recognition of the need to identify "standing grounds." In other words, some critical theorists argue that researchers and scholars should turn the critical lens on themselves, examining how their own perspectives have been shaped by gender, class, culture, and the historical moment, in order to understand the multiple influences on the questions they pose and the ways in which they pursue answers to those questions. This enterprise can admittedly swing too far into narcissism, but now that the academic "wars" over postmodernist thinking appear to have abated somewhat, many scholars seem more willing to be self-reflexive and examine the sources of their assumptions about the world.

The standing ground for our motivation to write about friendship and community has been constructed since the late 1960s, when, for a short time, we believed there might be a dawning "age of Aquarius," when all the peoples of the world would live together in peace and harmony. What dawned instead for us and many others in our cohort of leading-edge baby boomers were the challenges of adjusting to the demands of adulthood apart from the comforts of communal living among like-minded youth. Nevertheless, as we look back on the last thirty years of the twentieth century, we observe that in many ways we continued the "search for the good community," which was the title of a course we both took at Drew Theological School in 1971. It is instructive to see how that search was expressed through the many books we purchased and read through those years, beginning in the 1970s, a decade proclaimed by Tom Wolfe (1976) to be "the me decade." Of the many books we might note, two stand out because of the attention they received in the popular media for their critiques of the perils of excessive American individualism and the need to recover a sense of community.

The pages of our inexpensive paperback edition of Philip Slater's 1976 revision of *The Pursuit of Loneliness: American Culture at the Breaking Point* are yellowed, but today this work, having been scanned into the vast collection of Google books, can be read online. In this book, Slater laid out his argument that American culture was so enchanted by individualism that it frustrated the basic human desires for community, engagement with the social and physical environment, and dependence, by which he meant "the wish to share responsibility for the control of one's impulses and the direction of one's life" (9). Slater recognized the merits of American individualism in terms of the flexibility it afforded for change and adaptation to challenges, but he also understood the delusions at its core—delusions that rejected the fundamental interconnectedness among persons and between persons and their worlds. Though meant as a critique of economic and social structures supporting extreme individualism, Slater's book can also be read in light of the environmental movement that emerged in the late twentieth century and raised awareness of dynamic ecological connectedness. Slater's critics on the right argued that this book was just one more threat to the U.S. capitalist system and the rewards it provided to hard-working individuals, but Slater had no intention of calling for an end to individualism. Rather, he wrote, "far from trying to destroy our individualistic heritage, I'm only trying to collect on it. We're not going to stop being who we are—impatient of constraint, leery of group pressure, prone to doing our own thing—but we need to put aside our delusions. To believe that our fortunes aren't tied to everything that lives is a stupid and costly error" (169). In the 1970s, Slater was not thinking about how the fortunes of people with no memory loss might be tied to those who do experience progressive forgetfulness. However, his work is one example of the cultural critique of the late twentieth century that has influenced our examination of how persons who are living with dementia might contribute to vital communities of the twenty-first century.

About a decade after Slater released his revision of *The Pursuit of Loneliness*, another book appeared that generated widespread discussion in both academia and the popular media. *Habits of the Heart: Individualism and Commitment in American Life*, by Robert Bellah and colleagues (1985), took its provocative title from Alexis de Tocqueville, who chronicled his remarkable journeys through early American cities and towns in the two volumes of *Democracy in America*, published in 1835 and 1840. *Habits* analyzed the decline of forms of public life (e.g., involvement in voluntary organizations) that had been so richly depicted by de Tocqueville. Bellah and his coauthors described and documented how Americans in the late twentieth century had withdrawn from community commitments in favor of privatized pursuits of happiness and well-being. Most notable for those who studied American religious life was their description of a woman named Sheila, who described her religion as "Sheilaism"—a mixture of beliefs and practices she had blended herself. They observed that her approach to religion "somehow seems a perfectly natural expression of current American religious life, and what that tells us about the role of religion in the United States today" (221). They also pointed out that Sheila's religious individualism was not a new phenomenon of the mid-twentieth century but had roots in the earliest settlements of what became the United States. Through the country's history, it proved compatible with American religious pluralism.

Habits of the Heart should not be read as a simplistic rant against what some social commentators have called the "cult of selfhood." Rather, like Slater, Bellah and colleagues present a vision of how American individualism "is not to be rejected but transformed by reconnecting it to the public realm" (248). Although postmodern theorizing sometimes devolved into divisions sharply drawn by identity politics, it also taught us to think carefully about individual differences and the personal, social, and cultural shaping influences that create them. As we show in later chapters, recognition of the relational origins of personhood—including the personhood of people who are living with dementia—does not imply the rejection of respect for the attributes that make us unique, many of which are retained throughout the course of the dementia process.

The call for a renewed commitment to friendship and community balances recognition of the human need for separateness and privacy with the need for connection and public engagement. Another way that philosophers and psychologists have expressed this is in terms of the coexistence of the agentic and the communal. That is, human beings make decisions about their lives and exercise agency, but they do so within the context of relationality and community. Psychologist David Bakan (1966) described this as the "duality of human existence," and philosopher John Macmurray (1961) compared the "self as agent" and the "self-in-relation," concluding that the agentic self is constituted in relationship with other persons.

The creative tension between respect for individualism and the promotion of community health was lost at times during the 1990s, when culture wars erupted in many quarters in American society. Although Sheilaism could be found both in persons who had cut ties to religious congregations and in those who remained "in the pews," some critics saw it as the natural outcome of the spread of liberalism in politics and theology. Around the time when Robert Putnam first published his essay "Bowling Alone: America's Declining Social Capital" (1995), which he later expanded into a book, controversy was raging over communitarianism and its critique of exalted individualism.[11] Some laid the blame for the extension of the "me decade" through the end of the twentieth century on Americans' enthusiastic embrace of psychotherapy and popular forms of self-help, which seemed to be the outcome of psychology's triumph over religion.[12] Others blamed the "liberal church." Our professional roles in the last thirty years of the twentieth century—an academic psychologist and the senior pastor of large, liberal Protestant congregations—formed our standing grounds, from which we observed these arguments over individualism and the loss of social capital.

The View from the Lectern

It is not unusual for undergraduates to report hearing sociology professors state categorically that psychologists are blinkered in their refusal to pay attention to social dynamics. Well beyond the freshman lecture hall, psychology has the reputation—sometimes deserved—for its individualistic biases. Seeds of this reputation are planted early in American students' college careers, for those students in sociology classes are often also taking introductory psychology courses that reinforce the sociologists' opinions. For example, most of these psychology courses begin with a brief review of the history of the discipline. Although a few textbooks make passing reference to the pre-Socratic philosophers, and then Plato, and Aristotle, most proclaim that prescientific psychology (all thinking about behavior and mental life before the late nineteenth century) began with Descartes and his dualistic view of "the isolated individual understood as somehow definable introspectively, apart from any involvement in the world" (Swinton and McIntosh 2000, 177).

From Descartes, most introductory psychology texts move quickly from philosophy to territory psychologists inhabit more comfortably: the world of neurons and brain structures and various discrete psychological phenomena, like memory, motivation, and emotion. Only in the waning days of the semester will students discover that psychologists acknowledge that humans live in relationship to one another. In the chapters on social psychology that usually appear toward the end of texts, students learn about research on attitude formation, prejudice, and altruistic behavior. These chapters may also include research findings about close personal—often romantic—relationships. Friendship rarely appears in the indexes of these expensive, weighty textbooks, and when it is addressed, the discussion usually centers on variables that contribute to friendship formation, like proximity, similarity, and such personality characteristics as warmth, honesty, and loyalty.

Although the typical introductory psychology text includes a discussion of attachment theory in the section on infant development, the idea that the self is formed in interaction with other persons generally receives little attention. This may be due to the lag factor in textbook writing; although publishers assiduously claim to have updated each revision with the latest research findings, nevertheless paradigmatic shifts in disciplines are slow to seep into the books that introduce students to a field. This is certainly the case in psychology, which currently is undergoing what Ellen Berscheid (1999) calls "the greening of relationship science." She notes that psychologists search for explanations of behavior by studying individuals' temperament and personality with insufficient attention to the dynamic interactions of persons and their environments—which of course include other persons.

Berscheid argues that instead of viewing the individual as the unit of analysis, psychologists need to study the interconnections among human beings, interconnections occurring within particular environments at particular times. This view is neither revolutionary nor especially new, for there have been psychologists asserting this perspective practically since psychological research began. However, only recently has it begun to make its way into the mainstream of psychology.

Unfortunately, most psychology majors graduate with "encapsulated images of reality" (Royce 1973, 9), meaning that they have taken an array of courses, usually including social psychology, but they fail to see the big picture of how the various topics they have studied fit together. Their standing grounds are shaped less by "relationship science" than by their fascination with studies of the brain and nervous system and their dim understandings about genetic influences on various psychological characteristics. Thus, they go out into the world forever identified as having majored in psychology and uncritically ready to reinforce the biases they heard from their sociology professors opining about psychology's enchantment with individualism.

The View from the Pulpit

American congregations in the first half of the twentieth century would have been easily recognizable to de Tocqueville. Most were small, with fewer than 100 gathering for weekly worship. They were shaped and formed by the particular beliefs and practices of their denominational tradition but were often equally shaped by cultural and ethnic traditions. Any community resident could point out which Roman Catholic church was "the Irish church" or "the Polish church," and there might well be three Lutheran churches within blocks of one another, respectively shaped by Norwegian, Swedish, and German identities. One did not choose which congregation to participate in; one was born into the life of the congregation of one's parents and grandparents. It would be the setting for important markers in life's spiritual journey—for Christians, these were baptism, first communion, confirmation, marriage—before one was ultimately "buried from" that same church.

The church or synagogue was not only a spiritual center but also a social center, where members gathered to share communal meals and observe celebrations. Children belonged to the entire congregation, which shared in the task of instructing them in the tenets of faith and socializing them into the practices of the congregation. Older members were visible in a variety of leadership roles—deacon, trustee, teacher, or usher. Like any non-self-selected community, it brought together people who held a variety of political views, values, tastes, and interests. Inevitably, community members would "bump up against" one another from time to time, and relatively small matters—the color of a new carpet—could precipitate lively debate. If genuine community is, as one whimsical observer put it, "the place where the person you least want to be with always is," then the typical American congregation represented genuine community.

A variety of forces, many of them driven by free-market economics, brought significant change to American congregations in the postwar era. As the population became increasingly mobile, young adults were less likely to remain in the community of their childhood. Relocating to a new community required selecting providers for various services—a physician, a dentist—and a religious community became one more selection to make. Loyalty to a particular denominational tradition or ethnic heritage quickly faded as new criteria for making choices came to the fore. Which congregation makes me feel at home? Which has people my age who share my concerns, tastes, and interests? Where will our children receive the kind of religious instruction we wish them to have? Which congregation offers a youth program that will keep our teens coming back? A generation of Americans schooled in the ways of individualism came to see the selection of a spiritual home as one more consumer choice to make.

Economic forces were also at work that made it increasingly difficult for small congregations to remain viable. Growing numbers of women entered the workforce, diminishing the base of volunteers who had sustained the life of the congregation. As members sought more services and programs from the church, costs increased, particularly for staffing. Urban neighborhoods experienced "white flight," leading longstanding members to join new congregations in the suburbs where they now resided. Many small congregations shuttered their doors, while others merged with nearby parishes.

Even as neighborhood mom-and-pop stores were giving way to shopping malls and "big box" retailers, congregations began to make similar transitions. The baby-boom generation in particular became far more protean in seeking spiritual community, no longer feeling bounded by the religious tradition that had shaped and formed them. They wanted the best for their families, whether selecting a community, a home, an entertainment system, or a congregation. Churches began to define themselves as program-driven rather than centered in relationships within community. They sought to offer something for everyone, with a vast array of activities for all ages. They tailored worship services to the tastes of specific age cohorts—"traditional" worship for older members, "contemporary" worship for young adults, and "praise services" for teens. Generations were increasingly separated from one another.

These trends led to the birth of the *megachurch*, defined as a congregation in which four thousand or more people worship in a given week. With sprawling campuses surrounded by color-coded parking lots, such churches resemble the shopping malls near which they often locate. Their worship space typically looks like a movie theater, with individual seats replacing communal pews and people looking at the JumboTron screen rather than the actual speaker. Liturgy—"the work of the people"—is eliminated, sermons are replaced with simple "talks," and traditional hymns give way to upbeat praise music, conveying the message, This is not the kind of church service your parents forced you to sit through when you were a kid! Sharing in the life of such a congregation more closely resembles attending a sequence of performances and events than participating in the give and take of an actual community.

Interestingly, some observers believe that the trend toward megachurches may have passed its peak (as some say is also true about huge regional shopping malls). New forms of church, grounded in relationship and community, have been forming in recent years. They are assigned a variety of names—"emerging" church, new monasticism, new paradigm—but most value simplicity, informality, and "authenticity." They resist formal doctrine and eschew labels like "liberal" or "conservative." They place a primary value on the practices of hospitality and friendship. Among Jewish congregations, some Reformed and Reconstructionist synagogues are also promoting these values. Some people participating in these organizations live communally and hold at least a portion of their goods in common. It is a young movement, if it is a movement at all. Some view it as a response to the slickness of the megachurches and their perceived capitulation to consumerism and individualism, while others see in these new forms of congregational life a sincere effort to reclaim the central role of community for a new era. One dares to hope that the latter will prove to be true.

"Choking on truth"

Our particular standing grounds, formed from our experiences in academic psychology and liberal Protestant religious congregations, have repeatedly directed our attention to the excesses of desire for individual autonomy colliding with desire for submission to collective authority. Neither extreme can meet the coming challenges of an aging society in which some persons slip progressively into a world transformed by memory loss while others grow old with few noticeable cognitive changes. Thinking about aging and dementia calls for a critical examination of common assumptions about selfhood and about forming and nurturing friendships and good communities. This task will not be easy, for it must be undertaken against a backdrop of narcissism and fear.

At no other time in history have so many people been aging with such keen awareness of the perils of old age mixed with brash optimism about the promises of medicine and material wealth to eliminate those perils. Somewhere along the aging pathway, some people hope to spot a glorious fountain where they might sip the elixir of youth. Even without fantasies of finding that fountain, many have developed an image of what gerontologists call compressed morbidity, meaning that they will grow old experiencing high levels of health, psychological well-being, and social companionship until sometime in their nineties, when, after a short and relatively pain-free period of failing, they will cross gently over the edge of life to death. Unfortunately, however, this is not the way of death for most people in the twenty-first century. Rather, as Robert Kastenbaum (2004) says, we are both living longer and dying longer.

We once heard a respected geriatrician give a public talk about aging and dying today in which she asked how many in the audience hoped to live long lives. Every hand shot eagerly into the air. She next asked how many hoped to die of cancer, and the room fell silent and still. "Not cancer? So how many prefer to die of heart disease?" The silence became even deeper. "So you all are OK with frailty and dementia?" This image does not fit with the romantic image of compressed morbidity, and yet it is the one that the baby-boom cohort likely will face. Despite daily news releases proclaiming progress in identifying genes, proteins, environmental toxicants, and other possible triggers of various forms of dementia, none has been definitively identified and no cure appears to be on the horizon. We can Google our way to mountains of information about basic science and clinical research promising to prevent or cure the indignities of aging. But, even before the Internet made access to information so simple and sometimes overwhelming, we began to realize that we were, as Ernest Becker wrote in 1973, "choking on truth" (x).[13]

The marvelous and fearful discoveries of twentieth-century science could not eliminate death, though by seducing us with their promise to explain away all mystery, they cut us off from sources of cosmic and communal meaning (Moody 1986). In the twentieth century, aging, frailty, and death no longer occurred within a shared framework of transcendent meaning. Individual persons thus had to attempt to construct meaning on their own, an undertaking that works much better in times of economic security, good health, and plentiful social connections. However, the exciting challenge to create one's own worldview of meaning morphs into a heavy burden when the inevitable suffering and losses of aging can no longer be denied.

The baby-boom generation is living into the time of dementia. Honestly and courageously facing our anxiety and uncertainty about what that means might prepare us to create friendships and communities that relieve our despair over the impossibility of remaining "forever young." Some of us will experience progressive memory loss. But, as we show in this book, this condition does not have drain the experienced world of meaning. In communities of friendship where all persons—regardless of cognitive status—are valued, persons who have dementia can flourish. Given the opportunity, they can even teach the cognitively fit a few important lessons about growing old with grace.

CHAPTER ONE

Dilemmas of Dementia Diagnoses

"What is the difference between Alzheimer's and dementia?" This commonly posed question indicates the confusion and concern felt by the public about what has been called "today's most dreaded diagnosis" (Whitehouse and George 2008). In a later chapter, we address the anxiety—even the dread—more directly as we consider people anticipating the moment when they might have to hear the feared pronouncement (usually softened by the statement that the diagnosis is "probable"). For now, we introduce some basic information about several of the major forms of dementia and argue that the way dementia is usually portrayed limits our imagination and magnifies our fear.

This chapter describes what friends need to know about the progressive neurological conditions of old age that produce memory loss and confusion and suggests how they might move beyond images of loss and confusion while recognizing the suffering that comes with dementia. Without going into too much detail, we offer some basic information about what is known today, with the humble recognition that in just a few years, researchers and clinicians will no doubt change the labels and diagnostic criteria for many of these forms of dementia.

The very naming of the forms of dementia produces the illusion that they are immutable, but historical accounts reveal shifts in the ways researchers, clinicians, and the general public think about them. Moreover, lists of the symptoms of various forms of dementia tell only one limited part of the story about progressive memory loss. For this reason, the next two chapters move from the biomedical perspective to psychosocial, philosophical, and theological ways of thinking about the person who has dementia and the effects of brain changes on who we are and how others see us. Although we know that the labels and diagnostic tests will continue to evolve, persons who receive these diagnoses—however they are named—remain *persons*.

Because we are aware of the dangers of wandering so far into the thicket of biomedical descriptions of decline and deterioration that we lose sight of the human beings living with these diagnoses, we include short vignettes about people we have known. Science tells us how life looks from the outside, but stories give us an "inside view of life" (Birren 2001, viii). Students who endure classroom lectures accompanied by many wordy PowerPoint slides usually report remembering best the stories that illustrated the professor's points. People who listen to sermons week after week agree. Why? Gary Kenyon and William Randall (2001), two gerontologists who study older people's life narratives, say that "human beings are fundamentally storytellers and storylisteners. They not only *have* stories but *are* stories too" (4).

Three themes run through the brief stories we tell about people who are living with dementia diagnoses. First, the cognitive changes wrought by dementia shape their experience such that they live in the moment, a moment in which joy and love can be fully realized, even if accurate memories about the moment cannot be accessed after it has passed. Also, these moments are shared with others: family members, friends, and paid caregivers. Finally, these other persons have learned to appreciate those living with dementia just as they are; in other words, they make no effort to orient them to "reality."

Kinds of Dementia

The article in the newspaper asked readers to be alert for an older man who had wandered away from a residential facility. It offered a physical description of the man and the clothing he was wearing and closed with the words "he suffers from Alzheimer's and also dementia." Because Alzheimer's disease is a form of dementia, this description was akin to describing a missing pet as "a cat and also an animal." But given the general confusion about the various forms of dementia, it is also possible that the article was an awkwardly phrased but accurate description of a man who was experiencing more than one form of dementia, which is not uncommon. It is hardly surprising that many people are confused about the various forms of dementia, given how frequently terms are used incorrectly or interchangeably, even within the medical community.

There are many definitions of dementia, but one way of thinking of it is as a progressive decline in the abilities we usually categorize as cognitive or intellectual. These changes make various life activities—including interactions with other persons—increasingly difficult. Cognitive functions affected by dementia include certain types of memory, problem solving, abstract thinking, mathematical skills, judgment and decision-making, and language. However, we should not think of cognitive functions apart from a person's emotional life and the needs and desires that motivate behavior.

Failure to remember something important can be emotionally distressing. Inability to think clearly about the steps needed to accomplish a goal can disorganize behavior. Moreover, the location of changes in the brain that occur with various specific types of dementia can produce fewer memory problems but more difficulties regulating emotion and directing action. In other words, dementia can affect the whole personality, which encompasses the enduring, unique ways an individual thinks, feels, and acts.

Although a wide array of medical conditions can cause dementia-like symptoms at any age, our focus is on the progressive, irreversible neurodegenerative disorders normally associated with later life. Information about these disorders is widely available today in books and online resources.[1]

When reading information about the various forms of dementia, one must always keep in mind four important points. First, as ethicist Martha Holstein reminds us, "Whether the malady is a disease or an extreme version of normal aging, is interpretive as well as scientific and so not free of ideology and perspective" (2008, 260). Holstein wrote this sentence in a review of Jesse Ballenger's (2006) book *Self, Senility, and Alzheimer's Disease in Modern America: A History*. In this work, Ballenger tells the story of how American descriptions of "senility" in the late nineteenth century morphed into an eponymous name (Alzheimer's disease) for progressive memory loss in the twentieth century. It is a tale of profound sociocultural change, clashing scientific egos, and systematic public policy initiatives aimed at "fighting" a condition framed as a tragic loss of selfhood. Ballenger shows how we have created a culture (and an industry) of dementia, primarily by interpreting progressive memory loss solely in terms of changes taking place in the brain.

By focusing only on the brain, one can easily forget that brains enable the minds of unique, whole human beings. This leads to the second important point to remember when reading about various kinds of dementia: everyone who experiences dementia experiences it uniquely. In other words, as Downs, Clare, and Anderson (2008) put it, dementia must be viewed as a biopsychosocial condition. Yes, we can identify certain biological conditions that appear to be associated with forgetfulness and confusion. However, these conditions occur within individual persons with complex personal histories who live in particular sociocultural environments. Therefore, "the manifestation of dementia in any one individual . . . can only be understood by considering the interplay of neurological impairment, physical health, sensory acuity, personality, biography and past experience, relationships and social resources" (146).

The third point originated in writings about cancer and other diseases, but it applies to dementia as well: disease is not the same as illness.[2] *Disease* refers to pathogenic processes that occur within the body. Biomedical research attempts to identify the origin of these processes, the mechanisms that either keep them in check or produce their proliferation, and, of course, the interventions that can eliminate them. Thus, as we will see, various forms of dementia are said to be diseases because researchers and clinicians have identified changes in the brain that appear to correspond to changes in behavior and mental life. However, dementia is also an *illness*, which means that it is a uniquely human experience that produces not only physical and mental distress but also moral and spiritual distress. When people reflect on how a disease affects their sense of meaning and identity, they are experiencing illness. Illnesses have personal meanings, but these personal meanings are influenced by cultural meanings. Recall, for example, the time when no one could speak the word *cancer*. Persons who had cancer also suffered from the cultural meanings that stigmatized those with the disease. Similarly, today it is important to see how dementia is far more than disease processes in the brain; it is an illness with profound meanings for persons who receive the diagnosis, their families and friends, and the wider society of the twenty-first century.

Last, we must recognize the implications of the human need for naming. We name in order to understand, discuss, and, sometimes, to predict and control phenomena, whether we are talking about weather changes or human behavioral changes. We name, and we also order and categorize. Thus, we observe and name patterns in both weather changes and behavior changes. The increasingly fine-tuned names for various patterns of cognitive changes associated with dementia may create the illusion that we have indeed identified "real" disease categories. However, just a quick glance through the literature of the past twenty years shows that even in that short amount of time, the names have changed frequently.

Does this mean that new forms of dementia have suddenly emerged? No. We have simply acquired more observations, more data, and more technology that help us to "see" and define phenomena in a new way. In a provocative article on an emerging label we discuss later in this chapter—mild cognitive impairment (MCI)—Whitehouse and Moody (2006) argue that we are experiencing a "hardening of the categories" (11) with all this differentiation of brain pathologies. Paradoxically, they state that "new knowledge of neuroimaging and genetics has caused the boundaries among our dementia categories to become fuzzier rather than clearer" (21).

Aware of these four caveats, we now plunge forward and describe the most widely used names applied to the various ways progressive forgetfulness can be expressed. We do this because every day, people are acquiring these labels from physicians, neuropsychologists, and other health care professionals. However, these labels are very different from the ones we apply to other chronic conditions of later life, such as osteoarthritis. No one ever assumes that osteoarthritis attacks one's core being, but because we now so easily conflate selfhood and brain function, these names for the dementias are fraught with emotional meaning. Even though a person and family members may be relieved to "finally have a diagnosis," it is a diagnosis that has the potential to evoke deep despair and suffering because of the cultural burdens that shape dementia as an illness.

> When Ethel first heard the news a few years ago that she has "probable Alzheimer's disease," she was devastated. She says that was the worst day of her life, for she felt all hope drain out of life, like someone had pulled the plug on a bathtub full of water. Now, three years later, living with her husband (who also has the diagnosis) in an assisted-living residence, she looks back on that time and reflects on how much has changed. She is still able to drive locally, remains engaged with her church, and enjoys various group activities at the residence. She takes several medications prescribed to slow the progress of memory loss, but mostly she attributes her sense of vitality to other changes in her life. These were prompted by meeting a remarkable geriatric psychiatrist with a holistic, humane approach to working with people diagnosed with dementia. Ethel tells the story of going to hear him speak, and after his talk, spotting him talking with colleagues down a long hallway. She says she practically ran down that hall to say, "Dr. D——: You just gave me my life back!" He had spoken hopefully about healthy living, which includes a good diet, exercise, social engagement, opportunities to be creative, and the pursuit of spiritual practices like prayer, meditation, and communal worship. This doctor created the "Alzheimer's Center of Excellence," where his staff leads groups for people like Ethel. Together, several of the groups developed a poster featuring an image of the "Sun of Mindfulness" and the words *peace, love, joy*, along with lists of ways to be creative, still, relational, spiritual, and physically active. Ethel and her husband love going to the monthly group meetings, where they, like the other group members, walk into a medical office smiling, with happy anticipation of spending time there.

Alzheimer's disease (AD) is the most common form of late-life dementia, accounting for at least half of persons diagnosed with dementia. Including persons who have AD plus some other form of dementia increases that percentage to 75 percent.[3] Thus, it is hardly surprising that for many people AD and dementia have become virtual synonyms. AD typically emerges in later life, well after the age of fifty, although in a small number of cases, there are identified genetic markers associated with young-onset AD, the type originally identified by Dr. Alois Alzheimer in 1907.[4]

At least 10 percent of persons aged 65 have AD—often undiagnosed—and the risk grows significantly with advancing years, especially after age 85. AD most commonly presents initially through impaired short-term memory, which is why the "worried well" sometimes become anxious when they misplace their keys or glasses. As opposed to such normal forgetfulness, the person living in the early stages of AD has increasing difficulty consolidating new information and storing it in long-term memory. These memory difficulties begin to affect how a person conducts ordinary activities of life, such as remembering important dates, keeping track of finances, walking or driving familiar routes, and performing well-learned activities like cooking a favorite dish. Clinical testing can often (but not always) differentiate this form of memory impairment from the forgetfulness associated with normal aging, or even that which is associated with other neurodegenerative disorders. Such testing should always be conducted by a person who specializes in differential diagnoses, meaning that he or she can eliminate other possible sources of forgetfulness and confusion, such as medications, infection, malnutrition, and major depression, which could be treated.

AD is a progressive, irreversible, and ultimately terminal condition. When the brains of people with symptoms of AD are autopsied, pathologists find the characteristic plaques and tangles that Dr. Alzheimer observed in the brain of his famous patient, Auguste D. The plaques, which are formed from a sticky protein called beta-amyloid, accumulate outside the nerve cells (neurons) in certain parts of the brain and interfere with transmission of information among neurons. Over time, they show up in more parts of the brain, though the exact reason for their proliferation remains unclear. The tangles occur inside the neurons when tau proteins become twisted and tangled. The tau proteins act like a kind of scaffolding for the neuron, and they also form tiny pipelines—or microtubules—that transport nutrients in the neurons. The neuron becomes unable to function normally as these proteins become tangled, and eventually, it dies.

For many years, researchers have debated the chicken/egg question of which comes first, the plaques or the tangles. Currently, we do not know. On the other hand, what is clearer is that in addition to plaques and tangles, the brains of people with AD show signs of atherosclerosis, something else that Dr. Alzheimer noticed in Auguste D's brain.[5] Atherosclerosis happens when fat deposits build up in blood vessels, thus reducing the blood flow to and inside the brain. If neurons are deprived of blood, they are deprived of oxygen, with the result being cell death.[6]

As AD progresses, other cognitive processes besides memory are affected, including those associated with long-term memory, language, motor skills (dressing, using tools), visual skills (like recognizing objects), and the ability to integrate what one sees with the way one moves. The rate at which an individual journeys through the stages of AD varies. Some studies suggest that the average annual rate of decline in cognition is about 10 percent and that the illness usually leads to death within eight to ten years, but some persons who have AD live fifteen to twenty years, with periods in which the disease plateaus (Welsh-Bohmer and Warren 2006). It is important to note that depression may co-occur with AD and other dementias in as many as 40–50 percent of cases (Aniskiewicz 2007). Increasingly, clinicians are emphasizing the use of pharmacological treatments for depression, along with psychosocial interventions that improve overall quality of life—enjoyable social interactions, physical activity, and imaginative expression through storytelling and the arts.

Annie was an elegant woman in her early eighties. Her AD had advanced rapidly—four months earlier she was living independently and driving her own car, but now she resided in the dementia unit of a nursing home. Family members, concerned about her growing social isolation, were urging her to attend a musical performance in the facility's common room, but she declined repeatedly. Their presence was clearly causing her agitation—one family member suggested that they leave and return on another day. Then one family member, on impulse, tossed a small stuffed animal to Annie. Displaying the reflexes of a point guard, she snatched it from the air and tossed it to someone else. Soon a lively game of toss the tiger was in progress. Annie made as if to toss the tiger to her granddaughter, but did not release it. With a sly grin she repeated the motion several times, in the way we might tease a pet dog. When she finally released it, her granddaughter barked like a happy puppy. Annie, delighted that her joke was appreciated, broke into gales of laughter, with family members joining in. When the family left some time later, her daughter remarked in wonder, "I can't remember ever playing with Mom like that!"

Although AD has long been identified as the predominant form of dementia affecting older persons, until recently it was believed that vascular dementia (VaD) was responsible for the remaining cases. It is now suspected that *Lewy body dementia* (LBD, named after Friedrich H. Lewy, who in the early 1900s identified abnormal protein formations in the nuclei of neurons in parts of the brain), may be the second leading cause, accounting for 15–20 percent of all cases of dementia. Like AD, Lewy body dementia commonly occurs after the age of 60, but it is hard to be certain about prevalence because of its overlap with Parkinson's disease and AD. LBD progresses more rapidly than does AD, with the disease course usually lasting five years or less. Memory impairment is not always associated with the early stages of the disease, which is more likely to affect executive function (cognitive flexibility, concept formation, cue-directed behavior). Those who have LBD may fluctuate in cognitive function, attention, and alertness in cycles that last hours, days, weeks, or months. Visual hallucinations and depression often accompany LBD (in as many as half of cases), which has led to frequent misdiagnosis because these expressions resemble a number of psychiatric disorders (Welsh-Bohmer and Warren 2006).

There are days when Cynthia cannot distinguish between real and hallucinated visitors in her room. Sometimes the latter frighten her, and she screams horribly because a stranger has come into her room to spy on her. But one day her daughter arrived and found Cynthia calm and happy because she had just enjoyed a most delightful visit with her brother. She described all the topics they had discussed with each other. Her brother has been dead for more than six years. Cynthia's daughter listened with gratitude for her mother's good mood that day.

Joyce's LBD sometimes produces terrifying hallucinations of bugs and snakes crawling on her wheelchair. She shrieks for help when this happens. The CNAs who work at her dementia care residence have learned how to respond. They calmly come to her, acknowledge her terror, and gently say, "Oh, Joyce! We'll just move you to another chair." When they do this, Joyce smiles and is calm for a while. They keep two wheelchairs for her, and when she is having a bad day of hallucinations, they patiently transfer her back and forth.

Frontotemporal dementia (FTD) generally has an earlier age of onset (early fifties) than AD or LBD. Unlike AD, the risk of developing this dementia does not increase with advancing age. Estimates of its prevalence among persons who have dementia range from 4 to 20 percent. FTD can present in different ways, with some persons experiencing behavioral disorders and difficulties with executive function while others have language and semantic impairments. Persons who have FTD may exhibit disruptions in personality and behavior, including impulsiveness, loss of inhibition and social propriety, and lack of concern for personal hygiene. In its early stages it presents in a manner almost opposite to

AD—memory may be relatively unaffected while executive function, including social judgment, is profoundly affected (Welsh-Bohmer and Warren 2006).

> The man diagnosed with FTD was visiting with his son and another guest in a lounge at the skilled-care facility where he resides. Joe, who had been a pig farmer in younger life, was expounding with clarity and precision on things porcine (explaining why pork butt comes from the pig's shoulder, while ham comes from, well, the pig's butt). A young nursing aide entered the lounge and greeted Joe. He fixed his gaze on her clothing and asked, "What are you wearing under that outfit?" The aide gave him a mock slap on the shoulder and informed him that was none of his business. His son rolled his eyes and with a half-apologetic smile said to the guest, "You wouldn't believe how shy Dad used to be with women!"

Parkinson's disease (PD) is the most common movement disorder in older persons, commonly expressed through resting tremors ("pill-rolling"), rigidity, and slow movement. The cognitive impact of PD varies, with perhaps a third of persons who have PD meeting diagnostic criteria for dementia (PD-D). These persons may experience forgetfulness, slowing in thought processes, and difficulty maintaining attention. Depression and anxiety can accompany PD, and depression is said to be even more common among those who have PD-D (Cato and Crosson 2006).

> Al had lived with PD for many years, and he finally moved to a nursing home when his physical and cognitive conditions could no longer be managed at home. The chaplain at the nursing home had previously been a pastor in the community and had had a number of encounters with Al when he was younger. Al was a large, robust man in those days and had strong views on various religious matters. From time to time he would stop to visit the pastor's church to explain to him why his teachings were false. Now Al was thin and frail, drooled heavily, and could speak only in a whisper. When the chaplain stopped to visit, Al's eyes opened in recognition, and he haltingly raised his arms for a hug that extended for several minutes as he wept on the chaplain's shoulder. "Friend," he said again and again, "God bless you." Al no longer remembered his disagreements with the chaplain, only that he was a minister and that he was a friend who was present to him in his loneliness.

Alzheimer's disease, Lewy body disease, and frontotemporal dementia are usually broadly categorized as neurodegenerative dementias. Parkinson's disease, which may be accompanied by dementia and may also be linked with AD and LBD, is sometimes put in the category of "stable and slowly progressive dementias." This is a new, not yet universally accepted, way of categorizing certain dementias. Cato and Crosson (2006) place *vascular dementia* (VaD) in this group because it develops differently from AD, LBD, and FTD, and its pathology arises from changes in the large and/or small blood vessels in the brain. In VaD, one often observes a stepwise loss of function, often more obviously motor than cognitive and commonly ascribed to "ministrokes." The symptoms depend on where the blood vessels are blocked (ischemic damage) or where there has been hemorrhaging. VaD's relationship to AD is not clear, but it may co-occur in a third or more of all cases of AD (which contributes to disagreements about its prevalence). Typically, its onset is abrupt (although damage may accumulate silently before noticeable symptoms appear), and there may be relatively long periods of cognitive stability or even periods of partial recovery. The risk of developing VaD increases dramatically with advancing years (paralleling the risk of vascular events). Expressions of VaD may resemble those of AD (memory impairment) or PD (psychomotor slowing, loss of executive function).

> Tom's wife had known for some time that something was wrong with Tom. He managed life pretty well, but he was having trouble walking. At first she thought it was because of his hip replacement several years ago, but then she noticed his memory problems and difficulties in making decisions. Still, he was his usual pleasant, caring self, always eager to be with people and to help out when he could. Since retiring as a police officer in his town, Tom had volunteered for Meals on Wheels. A devoted volunteer, he had teamed with Mary for ten years. Mary happily describes how they came to be friends in that time of driving around delivering meals to homebound persons. However, Tom's driving was starting to worry her, especially after a close call. Recently, Tom went through a full diagnostic workup and received the diagnosis of vascular dementia. One result was that the doctor suggested he should no longer drive. Increasingly unsure on his feet, he was not able to carry meals to people's homes even if Mary did the driving. Not wanting let go of their friendship and knowing how much being a volunteer means to Tom, Mary calls him every week to report on the meal deliveries and keeps his name on the volunteer list.

These are simple descriptions, meant only to provide the current names of the most frequently diagnosed dementias and a few words about each. Although the initial hints of these various forms of dementia may differ, in all cases there are physical changes in the brain associated with the dementia—atrophy, loss of neurons (the nerve cells) and synapses (the connections between individual neurons), and the accumulation of plaques and tangles. Perhaps the strongest common element is the significant risk that the dementia will be accompanied by depression, whose symptoms may be masked and therefore left untreated. In many cases, when we believe we are observing the effects of dementia in a family member or friend, we are in fact seeing the symptoms of depression.

Cognitive Aging and Mild Cognitive Impairment

For all its wonders, the brain is an organ as surely as are the heart or the lungs, and like those organs it is not immune to the impact of aging. Just as athletes generally peak in physical ability in their early twenties, our cognitive-processing speed likewise reaches its maximum in early adulthood. But the skilled athlete may continue to improve in overall performance for an additional decade or more. The modest losses in absolute physical ability are offset by skills that become more refined through experience and greater emotional maturity. As we move through early adulthood and middle age, slowdowns in cognitive processing speed are compensated for by gains in judgment and wisdom. We acquire a greater context in which to place new learning, even if we may not absorb new information as efficiently and quickly as we did at nineteen.

As we age, our brains unavoidably undergo physiological changes. Good health habits—regular, vigorous exercise, proper nutrition, etc.—help maintain brain health as we age just as they help to maintain the health of other organs. But, we must not delude ourselves: despite the claims of purveyors of various nostrums and elixirs of youth, aging—including brain aging—cannot be halted or reversed. And as our brains age, even if they age in the healthiest way possible, cognitive changes will occur. We will have a bit more trouble paying sufficient attention to ensure that when we acquire new information, it can later be retrieved from memory. We will encounter that old tip-of-the-tongue phenomenon we have known most of our lives, only now the experience may evoke anxiety because of all the talk about dementia.

Healthy brain aging (that is, brain aging with no evidence of dementia) is generally described as "normal aging," a term we resist because it immediately labels those traveling the dementia road as "abnormal," even though journeying into dementia will be "normal" for as many of half of us if we live long enough. In many cases the boundary between normal aging and dementia is a gray and fuzzy area. It includes those who are functioning at a high overall level but are experiencing occasional memory lapses that create anxiety, as well as persons who will ultimately develop dementia. This boundary area, in which cognition is no longer regarded as normal relative to age expectations but in which daily functioning is not compromised to the point that a diagnosis of dementia is justified, has acquired the label "mild cognitive impairment" (MCI).

According to researchers at the Mayo Clinic, in Rochester, Minnesota, MCI describes memory impairment with no functional limitation, and it is viewed as prodromal—an early symptom of—dementia.[7] In other words, people said to have MCI experience difficulties with memory that exceed those found in most persons their age, and yet they continue to be engaged in their usual activities, managing their lives fairly well.

A key factor in the Mayo Clinic criteria for MCI is that individuals are aware that there has been slippage in memory functioning. One of the most noticeable behaviors is when they repeat the same question over and over, seemingly without awareness that they have just asked it and received an answer. Friends and family members may observe that conversations about things of little interest to the individual often seem to produce a kind of "fading out." However, as soon as the conversation returns to a familiar topic, the person can be quickly re-engaged. Although most daily activities continue in much the same way as they always have, certain tasks, like bill paying, which involves simple calculations, may become troublesome.[8]

> Harold gave a talk about living with MCI at a fund-raising dinner for the local chapter of the Alzheimer's Association. If his table companions had not known that he had been told he has MCI, they probably would never have guessed. Their conversation ranged over a number of topics, including the story of how Harold and his wife, both engineers, came to live in the United States after the Soviet Union had invaded Czechoslovakia. In his talk, Harold expressed deep gratitude for his wife's support and described his determination to live fully. An active participant in a brain and memory fitness group, Harold credited part of his sense of well-being to the friendships he had formed with members of the group.

Much MCI research focuses on estimating the percentage of persons who "convert" or "progress" to Alzheimer's disease and acquire the diagnostic label "early-stage Alzheimer's disease." Depending on the number of years of a longitudinal study, one finds figures like 12 percent of persons per year experiencing "conversion," 40 percent over two years, and up to 100 percent over nine and a half years (Modrego, Fayed, and Pina 2005). The 100 percent figure is part of what is driving some researchers to argue for revising diagnostic criteria in order to "capture the earliest stages of AD, including those individuals currently characterized as MCI for whom the cognitive impairment represents the earliest clinical symptoms of AD" (Morris 2006, 16).

Some who hold that most people with MCI progress to Alzheimer's disease argue that people should be diagnosed with Alzheimer's disease to begin with. However, a study published in 2009 argues that that conclusion may be too hasty. Researchers at the University of Leicester conducted a meta-analysis, meaning that they gathered a group of high-quality research studies and analyzed all the data together. In this case, they used forty-one different studies, some conducted in clinics where people were undergoing complete diagnostic testing and others done in the community, with less-rigorous testing. Their startling findings were that the annual conversion rate of people showing the characteristics of MCI as defined by researchers at the Mayo Clinic is only about 5–10 percent and that most people who have MCI will not develop dementia, even ten years after first noticing the annoying memory problems of MCI (Mitchell and Shiri-Feshki 2009). Some people even improve in their measured memory abilities. Observations like this have led one group of researchers to suggest that we have been far too inclusive in gathering older people with memory difficulties— including those who are not even aware of their problems—under the big tent of MCI (Purser, Fillenbaum, and Wallace 2006).

The Mayo Clinic criteria define subjective memory complaints as a key component of the diagnosis of MCI, while the European Consortium on Alzheimer's Disease decided that observations of memory problems could be provided by an "informant" (likely a spouse or adult child) even if the individual remains unaware of having difficulties (Portet et al. 2006). One study that followed people in Iowa for ten years concluded that people can have MCI without being aware of memory problems (Purser, Fillenbaum, and Wallace 2006). Whether a person "progressed" over that decade to a diagnosis of Alzheimer's disease seemed to depend not so much on the person's own recognition of memory problems or the worries of the informant, but rather the key component appeared to be difficulties in executive function, which are expressed via what are called "instrumental activities of daily living" (IADLs; Lawton and Brody 1969). Examples of this would be a person becoming confused when grocery shopping, having trouble following the order of adding ingredients to a recipe, mixing up the times for taking medications, or no longer being able to balance the checkbook.

On a parallel track with the tremendous increase in research on MCI is a growing critique of what Peter Whitehouse calls the attempt "to assign medical categories to what are a heterogeneous set of processes that affect our brains as we age" (2006, 87). While not denying the suffering of people with cognitive impairment, Whitehouse notes that "the stories we tell about brain aging can dramatically affect the quality of our lives and of our deaths" (87). These narratives can have devastating effects on people who receive the diagnosis, and on their families, when they are shaped around themes of loss of self and social meaning. Given our "hypercognitive culture" (Post 1995, 12), in which we equate personal value with memory and mental agility, these individuals and their families feel stigmatized (Katsuno 2005), fearful and uncomfortable with friends and relatives (Corner and Bond 2004), and embarrassed and ashamed (Frank et al. 2006).

If MCI is regarded as "the beginning of the end," it can plunge the person receiving the diagnosis into a pit of depression and despair. But it can also be a diagnosis that is constructive and hopeful if it is viewed as an opportunity to reach out for new resources—memory clinics, pharmacological interventions, exercise groups, workshops in the arts—that have potential for increasing the quality of life in the present and perhaps delaying the journey into dementia (if MCI is indeed a precursor to AD—a conclusion that is becoming suspect among some researchers).[9] It is also an occasion for renewing important relationships and pondering one's values and priorities.

MCI can be frightening because it points to a future filled with uncertainty. But uncertainty always defines the future, whether we acknowledge it or deny it. MCI does not define an inevitable future, but it encourages us to prepare for its uncertainty by living fully and thoughtfully in the present. Moreover, we have choices about how we interpret and cope with the aggravating memory problems that sometimes are given the MCI label.

Shifts in Thinking about Dementia

Although it is important to understand the distinctions among various neurodegenerative dementias, there is also danger in rushing too quickly to assign someone to a tidy, clinical category. AD, for example, can be expressed in a variety of ways and does not always progress in a predictable manner.

Peter Whitehouse, author of *The Myth of Alzheimer's*, argues that we should not speak of Alzheimer's as a disease at all but rather should view it as an expression of brain aging that occurs earlier and more precipitously in some persons for a whole host of biopsychosocial reasons. Although this is a minority perspective, Whitehouse is correct to note that aging affects all human brains, and it can be reductionist to assign a narrow clinical category to the manner in which such brain aging presents itself in a given person; too often it can lead us to see someone as a disease rather than as a person.

In other parts of the world, the broader term *dementia* is more likely to be used than *Alzheimer's* to describe someone experiencing progressive memory loss. To say "Bob is experiencing some dementia" or "Bob is living with dementia" permits us to remain open to the rich complexity of Bob's personhood and to view his life as full and vibrant while being sensitive to the challenges he deals with every day. To say "Bob has Alzheimer's disease" reduces him to a specific set of symptoms (even when such symptoms are not apparent). He is no longer a person, but a disease.

Whitehouse is not the only person starting to question our rush to hardened categories of diagnoses. In 2008, the *Journal of the American Medical Association* published an editorial called "Shifts in Thinking about Dementia." Its author, Vladimir Hachinski, of the Department of Clinical Neurological Sciences at the University of Western Ontario, argued that the very concept of dementia is outmoded and that trying to differentiate AD from VaD is an exercise in futility. Hachinski believes we need to start thinking about a continuum of cognitive changes in later life, some of which will produce the functional impairments we associate today with moderate and severe AD. He wrote: "Creating a dichotomy between dementia and nondementia ignores the spectrum of cognitive impairment. Converting soft data into hard categories fails to capture the complexity of the common coexistence and probable interaction of cerebrovascular and Alzheimer disease on the moving background of aging" (2172). Hachinski suggests that when medical care providers and aging persons collaborate to promote heart and vascular health, the age of onset of dementia can be delayed and prevalence reduced.

What is good for the heart is good for the brain, and the sooner this statement moves beyond being a slogan and transforms behavior, the sooner this shift in thinking about dementia can occur. In the meantime, however, we will probably see continued debate in the literature on the causes of Alzheimer's and the differentiation of one type of dementia from another. Arguments will also continue about whether clinicians can diagnose cognitive impairment in persons who are functioning pretty well in most aspects of their lives—impairment that some say represents the opening salvos of the slide into dementia.

Regardless of whether the future brings increasingly fine distinctions among forms of dementia, or whether many of the categories we currently employ are combined and redefined, people are still going to worry about their memory and their ability to remain mentally sharp as they grow older. Some of them may be given early screening tests as a part of routine medical care; others may wrestle with worry and finally make an appointment to "get checked out," often at the urging of family members. We suspect that people will be far more nervous about bringing the complaint of forgetfulness to their doctors than a bad cough. Thus, we need to look carefully at the psychological experience of receiving the diagnosis of dementia.

CHAPTER TWO

Receiving the Diagnosis

In the course of our lives we are likely to have many diseases and conditions diagnosed by a physician. We develop symptoms—a nagging cough, a swollen joint, persistent pain—that suggest all is not as it should be, and we consult our physician. Sometimes, we do this reluctantly or only because a loved one nags us into doing so. The physician may offer an immediate diagnosis or refer us for various tests.

At some point in the process, the disease or condition is given a name, and some form of treatment is suggested—surgery, medication, lifestyle changes—with the expectation that the disease will be cured, the condition will be healed, or, at the very least, will be managed in a manner that mitigates its impact on our quality of life. We expect our physicians to fix whatever is wrong with us.

If only the process of diagnosis were as straightforward in the case of cognitive impairment. As with any other condition, concerns about possible cognitive impairment begin with a set of symptoms that raise worries, either for the affected persons or for people who care about them. Perhaps he has gotten lost several times while in familiar settings. Perhaps she has been having difficulty remembering her own phone number or is forgetting to take important medications. Maybe in conversation with long-term friends he increasingly needs to pause to search for a familiar word. Or, most commonly, she asks a question that she asked just minutes earlier, or shares a bit of news, unaware that she shared the same information twenty minutes ago.

Often such symptoms of potential cognitive impairment develop gradually, so neither the person nor those around her can readily identify when "Mom's a little forgetful, but we all are sometimes" changes to "something is not right with Mom." We are adaptable creatures and develop work-arounds that mask minor problems with memory. The week's medications are placed in a daily reminder container, important phone numbers are entered into speed-dial, and an index card indicates the television channel of favorite programs. Family members and friends learn to listen to a repeated story without interjecting, "You just told me that!" Sometimes it is not until there is an incident that is genuinely frightening—Dad drives to the store to pick up his morning newspaper as he does every day, but this time he does not return and is found an hour and a half later miles from his destination with no sense of how he got there—that someone concludes that it is time to talk to the doctor.

Everyone around Dad, and likely Dad himself, has known that there was a problem greater than being a little forgetful, of course, but if many of us are prone to putting off a doctor's visit over a physical complaint for as long as possible, we are even likelier to procrastinate in consulting the doctor about cognitive concerns. Denial takes the form of a loving conspiracy: we all pretend not to see the issue for as long as we possibly can. For family members and friends, there is a desire to protect our loved one from being given a diagnostic label that we know will bring distress, anxiety, and embarrassment. For the person himself or herself, there is the fear that a medical diagnosis will make the condition real and that he or she will cross over the line from being a little forgetful to having a dreaded disease that marks "the beginning of the end." We know a woman in her eighties who counts backward from 100 by sevens several times each day because a friend told her that it is something people are asked to do when given "the test." She has convinced herself that as long as she can successfully pass her self-administered test, she cannot have dementia.

If we understand the diagnosis of cognitive impairment as a kind of death sentence, delaying that diagnosis as long as possible makes strategic sense, for that perspective too easily becomes a self-fulfilling prophecy. But if instead we view living with some degree of cognitive impairment as a next step in life's journey, one that does not preclude the possibility of living in a way that continues to be rich and fulfilling, then seeking diagnosis sooner can be helpful and positive. The better we understand what we are experiencing, the better prepared we will be to avail ourselves of resources that will enhance the quality of our lives. This is the reasoning behind the calls for early diagnosis.

Unfortunately, however, seeking a diagnosis may be a challenging process because, even as our society grows older, financial disincentives limit the number of physicians specializing in geriatric medicine. For most of us, the first step is an appointment with the family physician, who may or may not be knowledgeable about issues related to cognitive aging. It is not uncommon for the physician to act as a member of the loving conspiracy of denial. When a patient finally finds the courage to say, "I am having more and more problems with my memory," the physician may initially be dismissive of these concerns, responding, "We all get a bit forgetful as we get older." The physician may have his or her own fear of dementia to contend with, making it difficult to be objective, especially with a long-time patient.

Some physicians in general practice are reasonably well equipped to administer tests to identify cognitive impairment, but many are not. If the family practitioner does not feel competent to conduct a full cognitive evaluation, it is important to request a referral to someone who specializes in this area, even if that specialist is not conveniently located. In a proper evaluation, the clinician (most often a geriatric psychiatrist or geriatric neuropsychologist) will take the time to listen to the person being evaluated at length and develop some sense of who he or she is as a person. The clinician will make every effort to help the person to be comfortable and relaxed, because anxiety can have a negative effect on cognitive function. If the person wishes, a family member will be present to help in telling the story and to take notes on the information given by the physician. A complete medical history will be reviewed. The person will be asked about lifestyle, social network, and hobbies and interests. Other potential causes of the identified memory problems (including depression) will need to be eliminated. Various memory tests will be administered. In the end, the person may or may not receive a diagnosis.

It is much in keeping with our medicalized culture to desire a clear and definitive diagnosis—"Just tell me what it is, doc!" But "clear and definitive" can be an elusive goal in evaluating cognitive health, particularly if the clinician conducting the evaluation is meeting the person for the first time. A wise clinician will be cautious about tossing out a clinical label too quickly. If there is strong evidence pointing to Alzheimer's disease, the clinician may make that diagnosis; many will label it as "probable Alzheimer's."

In the best scenario, the focus of the discussion after testing will be on both psychosocial and pharmacological interventions that may help with memory function and general quality of life. In other words, using the differentiation of disease and illness we made in Chapter 1, the best clinicians speak to the person experiencing an illness about the ways a disease was diagnosed and how it might be addressed holistically by the person with the diagnosis and close family members and friends. The clinician may offer information about a memory center in or near the local community that offers support groups, classes, and activities designed to help enhance or retain memory function. People may receive recommendations of helpful books and Websites. The goal is for the person being evaluated to feel comforted by knowing that support will continue from the clinician and other caring professionals in the community.

In an ideal world, a person who arrives for diagnostic evaluation in a state of fear and anxiety will leave feeling far more optimistic about the future. Sadly, this remains a minority experience. In too many cases, the evaluation is brief and impersonal. A clinician with a full appointment schedule conducts a cursory examination, asks a few questions and pronounces (often to the spouse or child, rather than to the person) "Your mother (father, husband, wife, sister, brother) has Alzheimer's." (Note that this conversation would most likely not include the statement "your *friend* has Alzheimer's" due to legal protections for patient privacy that prevent unrelated persons from being included in medical examinations.)[1] We have heard many stories of persons who were handed a brochure from the local Alzheimer's Association, given a prescription for one of several types of drugs that may slow the progress of forgetfulness, and sent on their way to cope with a terrifying new way of living.

How will people respond to this news? The first thing to remember in thinking about possible answers to this question is that responses evolve over time. In other words, receiving the diagnosis is not an event but a process. How the process unfolds will depend on many factors related to the individual as well as to his or her social environment.

One interesting study followed couples over the course of several months. Researchers interviewed them two weeks after the diagnosis was made and again after twelve weeks. People varied in their responses, with some actively trying out new ways of "making the best of things" while others struggled to accept why certain important aspects of their lives had changed—the freedom to drive, for example. A few couples made some significant life decisions, with one couple getting married after many years of living together. Others focused more on the emotional adjustments they were making together. Overall, the researchers were impressed with people's attempts to cope, although they thought that perhaps the participation in the research itself—interviews with people who cared about how they were responding—might have been one factor that reduced some people's feelings of devastation (Vernooij-Dassen et al. 2006).

Researchers are starting to develop models that can help us understand who will say, "Call Dr. Kevorkian," and who will say, "OK, now what do I do to go on living well?" We can take two related approaches to understanding people's reactions. One comes from several decades of research on stress and coping, and the other is emerging from research specifically focused on dementia.

Stress and Coping

The idea of "stress" originated among seventeenth-century engineers who were trying to figure out how load affected objects (like bridges, for example). It was adopted in the early twentieth century to refer to external forces that strain individuals (just as a heavily loaded cart strains the animal pulling it and the bridge it is crossing). However, beginning in the 1960s, psychologist Richard Lazarus argued that the engineering analogy does not work for human beings for one important reason: we have the ability to appraise situations that might be described as stressful. We can think whether we have ever encountered similar situations in the past, how we dealt with them, how threatening they are to us now, and what we plan to do in response.

Sometimes, under some conditions, both physical and environmental, a particular "load" will produce a lot of stress because the individuals experiencing it perceive that they have few resources to deal with it. Take, for example, having an ordinary head cold. With no approaching work deadlines, a whole weekend to stay indoors on the couch with a good book, tea, and tissues, a person might not experience the load of infection with rhinovirus to be particularly stressful. On the other hand, experience the first juicy symptoms of a cold while on an airplane that arrives late to a city where you are giving a big, important talk the next morning, and you might come up with a very different appraisal.

Lazarus made an important distinction between types of appraisal. Primary appraisal means our assessment of the threat. How bad is it? Secondary appraisal refers to our assessment of the resources we have available to cope with the threat. These resources are either internal or external and can take physical, psychological, social, or spiritual forms. Going back to having a head cold, a person's primary appraisal might be "it's not so bad; I've had worse." Secondary appraisals might include this inner monologue: "Overall, I'm healthy; I'm in a good place psychologically; my friend is bringing chicken soup tonight; and in the cosmic scale of things, a head cold is of little significance." On the other hand, that person heading to a big meeting might also say "it's not so bad; I've had worse" but could have fewer resources: the cold comes just as he has healed from a broken ankle, this big meeting could be the turning point in a career, an important relationship just ended, and all alone in an unfamiliar city, he feels a sense of existential despair.

Think of the many ways people might appraise the experience of becoming confused while driving a familiar route, being unable to balance a checkbook, forgetting a frequently used recipe, repeatedly having adult children say "Mom, but I already told you that," getting mixed up about taking medications, and so on. We cannot make a prediction because individuals will interpret these situations differently. Some will experience an acute threat; others will not. Some will be secure in calling on inner and outer resources; others will feel they have nowhere to turn. Lazarus described the personal significance of potential threats and challenges as reflecting their "relational meaning" (Lazarus and Lazarus 2006).

During the decades at the end of the twentieth century, Lazarus and his colleagues gathered considerable evidence demonstrating the dynamism of these forms of appraisal and their central role in affecting how people cope. These researchers identified two particular ways of coping, which they called "problem-focused" and "emotion-focused" (Folkman and Lazarus 1980).

Some people, in some situations, can directly address threats and deal with them, thus solving problems by changing the situation. They can make a plan and carry it out to relieve stressful circumstances. But stress is not always so easily eliminated or controlled. Then people employ ways of coping that enable them to change how they feel about the situation. Some of these responses are maladaptive, as when people self-medicate with drugs and alcohol as a way of "killing the pain." Other emotion-focused responses are more adaptive, such as when people adopt strategic reinterpretations ("this really isn't so bad") or compare themselves to others ("they've got it much worse than me"). Humor can also be used to deflect painful emotions. Sometimes people call this denial, but we need to be cautious about casually tossing out that accusation because there are circumstances under which denial can have a positive relational meaning. Consider this example:

> When Roger was struck by a severely damaging stroke in the left hemisphere of his brain, which left him paralyzed on one side, confused, and unable to speak, his wife described him to family members as having encountered "a little problem." A little problem? No, this was a major, life-changing event! However, in the face of such turmoil, the only way she could hang on from moment to changing moment for a few days in the intensive care unit of the local hospital was to say he had a "little problem." Later, when he was moved to a rehabilitation facility, where she faithfully visited and participated in his therapy, she slowly was able to recognize that their problem was not little at all.

Religious faith is sometimes categorized as being a form of emotion-focused coping. It can help people change their interpretation of stressors or their assessments of their personal and social resources for coping. Thus, psychologists have viewed prayer and meditation as ways in which people regulate their emotions. Although religious beliefs and feelings are often cited as the most common resource for coping among older adults (Koenig, George, and Siegler 1988), some forms of religious coping are not effective and may be more harmful than helpful.[2] Although psychologists usually put religion into the emotion-focused coping category (which some mistakenly assume is less effective than the direct, active, problem-solving approach), we suggest that support offered by faith communities to people struggling with threats and challenges can sometimes take the form of problem-solving. Laura and Phil showed us how this might happen.

> Laura cared for Phil for several years as he slipped deeper into the confusion of Alzheimer's disease. Finally, she was unable to meet his physical needs at home, and he moved to a skilled-nursing facility. This was an extremely difficult decision for Laura to make. One of the things she most missed was the small dinner parties she and Phil had hosted for many years. Four friends from Phil and Laura's church stepped in and helped her solve this problem. Once a month, they brought food, a tablecloth, and fancy serving dishes to the nursing home. Phil couldn't talk much to participate in the conversation, but his smiles and hand gestures communicated his pleasure. For Laura, these evenings were deeply meaningful and delightful opportunities to get together with caring friends. She also felt that she was doing her part to help reinforce positive attitudes about dementia and nursing homes for her friends.

Do We Want to Know?

Today, it is possible to determine if a person has inherited a rare genetic trait that has a high probability of producing the kind of Alzheimer's disease that first becomes noticeable in middle adulthood. Although the changes in the brain—the sticky plaques outside of the neurons and the tangles inside the neurons—may be similar in persons with this young-onset, familial Alzheimer's disease and those who develop symptoms in their seventies or later, the latter, "garden variety" Alzheimer's disease cannot be definitively predicted through genetic testing.

In considering the complex biological and ethical issues raised by genetic testing, we need to remember that genes work in concert with the environment, which includes the physical world and the social world. Consider, for example, the environmental factors that could have contributed to the risk factors identified in a recent study of older persons (Barnes et al. 2009). Participants, whose average age was 76, were assigned points depending on the presence of a particular gene form (the apoliprotein E4 allele), along with their age, body mass index (BMI), cognitive test performance, MRI evidence of brain abnormalities, atherosclerosis (thickening of the arteries), history of bypass surgery, speed of physical responses, and amount of alcohol consumption. The number of points they received was related to their probability of being diagnosed with dementia six years later. Although all the risk factors can be viewed strictly from a biomedical perspective, most can also been seen as reflecting choices people make and resources available to them in the environments they have experienced since birth.

So far, it is not possible for one of the "do it yourself" gene-testing kits to predict dementia risk,[3] and many dementia researchers argue that this can never happen because of the complex relationships between persons and their environments from infancy onward. Nevertheless, we have no doubt that some people will continue to express a kind of genetic fundamentalism, believing that genomic science can resolve all of life's uncertainties.

As we noted in Chapter 1, even without a definitive genetic test, we have today achieved the ability to diagnose "probable Alzheimer's disease" with some certainty by using a battery of cognitive tests and brain imaging. Thus, increasingly, people are sitting in doctors' offices, hearing the dreaded words pronounced: *probable Alzheimer's disease*. Rebekah Pratt and Heather Wilkinson (2003) conducted what they called the "Tell me the Truth" study to find out more about people's reactions to hearing these words. They suggested that there are two important contributors to people's reactions to receiving the diagnosis: their desire and ability to know the diagnosis, and the social context in which they live. Thus, like Lazarus, they do not view the experience of stress, or the response of coping, as lying solely within the domain of the individual.

Pratt and Wilkinson begin by noting that throughout their lives, some people "hide their heads in the sand," retreating from bad news of all kinds. This is the way they have coped in the past with life's challenges, and there is every reason to believe that this is how they will respond to receiving a dementia diagnosis. Others, however, cope best when they know as much as possible about the challenge they are facing. (Of course, today with so much information readily available on the Internet, people can quickly access a lot of information, not all of which will be helpful or accurate.) Thus, some people have a strong desire to know the diagnosis. However, because of the progressive nature of dementia, they may not be able to understand what the physician or psychologist is saying about the diagnosis, particularly if this conversation is not sensitive to the intellectual capacity and emotional state of the individual.

The other part of Pratt and Wilkinson's model describes the social context in which people receive the diagnosis. It can influence their response because it includes the reactions of family and friends, the attitude of the doctors or psychologists who have conducted the diagnostic procedures, the social stigma attached to dementia, and the availability of support from others, including community programs devoted to maintaining life quality for those who are living with dementia.

Pratt and Wilkinson's model can be pictured like this:

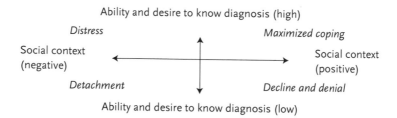

People who want to know all about the diagnosis and the expected outcomes, and who have the ability to take in this information but who have family members and friends who are fearful or even angry about the diagnosis, will probably experience considerable *distress* and conflict. They might want to know, but they feel forced to protect others from the knowing.

On the other hand, if the individual does not want to know and has loved ones in complicity with that position, there may be a kind of *detachment* from the whole issue. These persons may not even come for a diagnosis in the first place because even though they may be aware of some changes in their ability to remember, neither they nor their social partners want to face up to the potential diagnosis.

People who have the combination of a high ability and desire to know, along with a supportive social environment, can make the most of various coping strategies because they have personal resources (e.g., a positive attitude and the ability to collaborate in decision-making about day-to-day life and future planning) and support from other people to face the diagnosis squarely and determine the best way to make life good. Below this quadrant of *maximized coping* falls a quadrant formed when a person has low desire to know the diagnosis because the progression of confusion and forgetfulness has challenged the ability to have enough self-reflection to understand it. Pratt and Wilkinson call this *decline and denial*. Note that this quadrant includes a supportive social environment. Family members and friends do not hesitate to show their love and care for the individual who has become unable to engage actively in making sense of the diagnosis.

In summary, Pratt and Wilkinson's model says that a person's reaction to experiencing memory problems and receiving the diagnosis of Alzheimer's disease or some other medical category of dementia depends on the individual and the people surrounding him or her. As Richard Lazarus repeatedly argued in his work on stress and coping, responses to challenges like having memory problems and making decisions about whether to seek a diagnosis depend on a complex interaction between personal characteristics and the situation (which, of course, includes other people). Complicating the application of the Lazarus stress and coping model, and the Pratt and Wilkinson model, is the fact that human beings live in time. When considering how people respond to the dementia diagnosis, we always need to factor in the progressive nature of the changes wrought by dementia. Whether a person is in the early or the late stages of dementia can shape both the individual's reactions and those of other people.

What Do the Stages Mean?

One of the defining characteristics of our human mental activity is that we organize information into categories that we often order by ranking: from most appealing to least appealing, from strongest to weakest, from best to worst. We do this with fruits and vegetables, with people, and, of course, with diseases. Our categories and rankings give us a sense of control that is often useful as we make our way in the world, faced with so many decisions. We can even rank the types of decisions we need to make, from those that have few long-term effects to those that are literally a matter of life or death.

The notion of stages is implicit in the very idea of dementia, for it describes a progressive loss of memory and other cognitive functions. Go to nearly any Website on Alzheimer's disease or other dementias, and you will find descriptions in terms of time (early to midstage to late) or strength and severity (mild to moderate to severe).

A well-known stage model—the Global Deterioration Scale (GDS; Reisberg et al. 1982)—defines seven stages, beginning with "no cognitive decline." We find it odd that a person who shows no clinical characteristics of dementia and normal scores on various psychological tests of cognitive function is still categorized as having "stage 1" disorder.[4] On the other hand, perhaps this can be viewed as a great leveler, eliminating the "us" versus "them" problem arising when one individual has a diagnosis and another does not. People often ask "what stage?" when they hear that a friend or family member has received the diagnosis of Alzheimer's disease or some other dementia. Perhaps they should also say, "Well, I'm still at stage 1, but I may eventually join you at stage ____."

Being given a diagnosis and a stage classification can comfort some people, for despite the progressive nature of dementia, the actual rate of progression is variable. It may be slowed by interventions like pharmaceuticals or by a change in diet, exercise, social engagement, or cognitive stimulation. The rate of progression also depends on a person's "reserve capacity," meaning the strengths built up over a lifetime of learning, eating a healthy diet, staying fit through exercise, and having meaningful, caring relationships with other people.

The issue of stages of dementia raises the question of people's awareness of their condition. Often, doctors treat awareness as a biomedical symptom, considering more awareness of difficulties to be evidence that the person has just begun the journey into dementia, while lack of awareness signals the later stages. Linda Clare's (e.g., 2003) psychosocial approach stands in contrast to the biomedical one, for she argues that people who have dementia make choices about how they present themselves, both to preserve their sense of who they are and to protect those close to them.

Even when people get to the later stages, passing over the boundary from "early dementia" to "moderate," "moderately severe," or "severe dementia" (Reisberg et al. 1982), they are still capable of talking about their lives and their problems remembering and thinking. For example, Linda Clare and colleagues interviewed eighty people who were living with moderate to severe dementia in a long-term care residence. All of them showed some forms of awareness. They talked about having memory problems and having to rely on other people. They described their feelings of loss and isolation from family and familiar surroundings. Overall, despite expressing frustration about some aspects of their daily experiences, they showed themselves to be actively coping by "making the best of things" and by reminding the interviewers of their past identities (Clare et al. 2008a, 2008b).

These studies are important because they reveal that persons who often show considerable confusion and memory loss can still demonstrate that they are aware of their environments, the feelings of their bodies, and their emotions. Many were also able to reflect on their experiences of being confused about time, place, and the identities of other people.

In her studies of people who have not yet progressed so far as to need residential care, Clare and colleagues identified a continuum of active coping responses, ranging from efforts to maintain life as it has always been to deliberate efforts to adjust to the difficulties produced by progressive forgetfulness. They call one end of this continuum the "self-maintaining" approach and the other end the "self-adjusting" approach. They do not claim that one is preferable; in fact, they note that over time, people show both reactions (Clare, Roth, and Pratt 2005). People with memory loss work hard to normalize their situations despite the challenges of their cognitive problems, but they may also make some practical changes in the ways they manage their lives and their relationships.

> Frank has been diagnosed as having early-stage dementia for about six months. He lives alone in a neat ranch home decorated with many pictures of his sons, their wives, and a newly adopted granddaughter. His wife died about two years ago, and he is now dating a woman he calls his "lady friend." He says, "She gets me enthused about things." One day, while undergoing a physical, he mentioned that he had been forgetting things. His doctor sent him for a battery of neuropsychological tests resulting in his diagnosis. He said he was not surprised, as his father "had it" and his two sisters "have it" now. He has started attending a "memory fitness" group on the recommendation of his geriatric psychiatrist. He is still driving, but he worries about losing his driver's license even though he recently passed a road test "with flying colors." He believes that his medications, new approach to diet and exercise, volunteering at a local food bank, the memory fitness group, and the support of his sons and lady friend are all making a difference and that he hasn't experienced himself as "getting any worse."

The work of Linda Clare and many other researchers who take the time to listen to people who have dementia reveals much about their humanity. Unfortunately, sometimes we allow the scientific-sounding diagnostic categories and descriptions of stages of deterioration to define the story we tell about them. This quickly becomes a story of otherness, which creates barriers to meaningful relationships. However, there is a new story being told about dementia, a story about personhood and identity. It is woven through much of the psychosocially based literature on dementia published since the 1990s. On a parallel track, an old, old story about personhood is being retold by philosophers and theologians.

CHAPTER THREE

Personhood

On several hot August days in 1998, a group of people who described themselves as "change artists" met in a continuum-of-care retirement community in Oshkosh, Wisconsin, to continue a discussion that had begun the year before in Rochester, New York. Some of these folks remembered the 1960s and the VW buses they used to drive from concert to concert. Now middle-aged and in respectable positions as nursing home administrators, social workers, psychologists, and doctors, they imagined getting on a bus and driving around the country, going from town to town to proclaim a new way of thinking about community and personhood and about aging and dementia. Nursing home residents, they said, should be given choice and control over as many aspects of their lives as possible. Every person, including those who have the most advanced dementia, has potential for growth. Intentional community formation is essential to combat the isolation, boredom, and helplessness that are too prevalent in long-term care facilities. This gathering of "nursing home pioneers" at times felt subversive, for its goal was nothing less than changing the culture of aging and nursing home care in America.[1] Over and over, people talked about the huge impact of a small book that was still rather hard to come by in the United States. Written by British psychologist Tom Kitwood (1997), *Dementia Reconsidered: The Person Comes First* gave this group of pioneers a conceptual structure that undergirded their plans for radical reform of senior services and nursing home care.

Tom Kitwood taught that dementia care must be grounded in a relational view of personhood, which he defined as "a standing or status that is bestowed upon one human being, by others, in the context of relationship and social being. It implies recognition, respect and trust" (1997, 8). In his book, Kitwood offered many examples of the "old culture" of dementia care, in which persons were treated like warm objects (or worse yet, as "vegetables") occupying space, needing occasional feeding and cleaning and care for medical problems like infections or broken bones. The "old culture" dehumanized not only persons who had dementia but also those who cared for them because of the contagious nature of stigma.[2] It goes like this: If I am caring for a person viewed as having no value, then how can my work, and my personal investment in it, have meaning and value? If my hard work has no meaning and value, do I, as the worker, have any meaning and value to my community and the larger society?

Kitwood's work helped to transform perceptions of persons who have dementia and the care they receive. It also inspired a new way of thinking about how organizations should value the persons employed to provide care. In other words, changing the culture of dementia care requires a change not only in how the person who has dementia is viewed but also in the treatment of CNAs (certified nursing assistants) and others who represent the front line of dementia care. Their personhood also must be affirmed with "recognition, respect, and trust."

In the late 1990s, Kitwood's teachings about personhood and a new culture of care took root in a few nursing homes and other residences for older adults who are living with dementia. The transition to the new culture is fraught with many challenges from residents, families, and staff, for the idea of "person-centered care," which accompanies these changes, is often hard to implement. Some residents, family members, and nursing home staff prefer the old culture, in which everyone has a strictly defined role and authority for decision-making flows from the top down. The person-centered approach to care offers residents as many opportunities for choice as their interests and cognitive and physical skills allow. The documentary film *Almost Home* shows how the change to person-centered care at a continuing-care retirement residence in Milwaukee invites people living with various degrees of memory loss to make choices ranging from whether to have toast or cereal for breakfast, to preferences about accompanying family members on an outing.[3]

Almost Home vividly portrays the conflicts that arise when the ideals of person-centered care meet the realities of everyday life in a complex organization devoted to providing high-quality nursing care, assisted living, and independent living. For example, in one scene, a nurse plainly states that the old way of passing out medications—using a cart pushed up and down the hallways—was far easier. However, the administrator leading the organization through this change in its culture argues that people do not have big carts rumbling through their homes, so they should not have them in this new home. Medications should be stored in locked cabinets in each resident's room. The nurse argues that residents do not stay in their rooms; they wander freely about the facility, and thus the nurses are forced to "chase them down" to give them their medications. Another challenge in the change to person-centered care arises from the notion that all staff members (including administrators) should be able to give various kinds of care to residents. The old culture had strictly defined job parameters, but in the new culture, if an employee passes a room with a call light lit, he or she should stop in to see how help can be given. This kind of change does not come easily, and the film insightfully portrays the struggle to fit the ideals of the new culture with the habits and expectations of the old culture.

Names have power, and because they do, they are often the source of controversy. For example, soon after "person-centered care" entered the lexicon of gerontology, some people working with older adults, primarily in residential care, argued that "resident-directed care" was preferable both descriptively and prescriptively. However, reflecting on Kitwood's relational definition of personhood, some then stepped up to argue that perhaps we ought instead to be talking about "relation-centered care." For example, an article coauthored by researchers from Sweden and the United Kingdom showed how public policy in both countries had adopted the language of person-centered care, which, paradoxically, ended up having "a distinctly individualistic focus" (Hellström, Nolan, and Lundh 2005, 17), which ignored interdependence.

We may begin with debates over labels, but the discussion quickly moves to fundamental assumptions about what it means to be human and to live together in community. Can we creatively work with the tension between maintaining recognition of the uniqueness of each individual and at the same time acknowledge our interdependence? Organizations like the one portrayed in *Almost Home* promote the option of "independent living," but what does this really mean? These questions have taken on new meaning in this time of increasing numbers of persons diagnosed with dementia. As we assert throughout this book, progressive memory loss and confusion challenge us to think carefully about selfhood and community—about dependence, independence, and interdependence—in the twenty-first century.

Culture change. Personhood. Relationality. These terms now roll easily off the tongues of many people working in organizations that serve older adults. Sometimes, they are mere window-dressing—clever ways of marketing what is essentially the same old hierarchical, top-down decision structure that leaves little room for elders or those caring for them to make choices or exercise any control over their daily lives. But, before we permit ourselves to become too cynical about this, we should acknowledge that a real sea change has occurred not only in gerontological practice but also, more generally, in the social sciences.

It seems that everyone these days is talking about community—"no man is an island"—and the image of human identity as a compounding of multigenerational relationships, beginning with the earliest ones, with parents. Recall that in the Introduction to this book, we noted that psychology had been criticized in the past for its limited focus on autonomous individuals. Although this might have been true in some quarters in the mid-twentieth century, that time has passed. We now have a robust (though still controversial) subfield called "evolutionary psychology," which examines various individual behaviors in light of their effects within social groups. Increasingly, social scientists and neuroscientists are collaborating on studies that fall into a category called "social neuroscience," which begins with the proposition that the brain is essentially a social organ (Cacioppo et al. 2007).

Time Out for Monkeys and Children

Why monkeys? This is not a detour through the theory of evolution, but rather a description of studies of infant rhesus monkeys conducted in the 1950s by Wisconsin professor of psychology Harry Harlow. Though severely criticized now for the way the young monkeys were treated, this research poignantly revealed the power of emotional bonds, especially under threatening or uncertain conditions. Harlow and his students claimed they were studying love in the infant monkeys. They removed the babies from their mothers shortly after birth and placed them in cages with two "surrogate mothers," which were actually wood-and-wire contraptions. One was covered in terrycloth and the other was covered in chicken wire. Though fed from a bottle poking out of the "wire mother," the babies developed no discernable emotional attachment to it. Rather, they spent nearly all of their time clinging to the "cloth mother." When Harlow placed a "fear object" (a clanking flashing robot) in the cage, the infants fled to the cloth mother. In a large empty box (called an open field) with no place to hide, the monkeys also cowered on the "cloth mother." Occasionally, they ventured away to explore a bit, only to return immediately if the environment was even slightly disturbed by a sound or light.[4]

Why children? Harlow's work confirmed in a nonhuman species what British psychoanalysts Rene Spitz and John Bowlby observed in human children separated from their parents. Spitz famously described children living in orphanages where, despite good physical care, they suffered a profound lack of emotional attention. They lost weight, withdrew from any engagement with others, and some even died. Bowlby knew about Spitz's work, as well as the studies of the ethnologist Konrad Lorenz, who had described how newly hatched ducklings became imprinted to the first moving thing they saw, which as a widely reproduced photograph showed, often was Lorenz himself.

Combining the observations of young animals and young humans, John Bowlby developed attachment theory, which he claimed described an inborn biological bonding system (Bowlby 1969–80). As anyone who has spent time with children knows, they seek their parents when they are distressed. The parent represents a safe haven to retreat to under conditions of threat, as well as a secure base for exploring the surrounding territory when the child is confident of the parent's steady presence. Like Harlow's baby monkeys, young children need to snuggle up with someone to whom they have become emotionally attached, especially when they feel uncertain or threatened.

Bowlby's theoretical and clinical work inspired psychologist Mary Ainsworth and her colleagues to develop a laboratory test that assessed various types of attachment children formed with their parents (Ainsworth et al. 1978). Working with children as young as two, Ainsworth could see that some were securely attached to their mothers (in the 1960s, few studies paid attention to fathers), but others were insecurely attached. Either they seemed anxious about their relationships and not quite sure if their mothers did offer safety and security, or they avoided going to their mothers for succor and support. These attachment styles are not immutable, but many studies have indicated that they can persist through adulthood.

Psychologists have now been studying attachment in children and adults for more than fifty years. Despite some disagreement about how to measure it and how to describe different forms of insecure attachment, there is solid consensus about the fundamental precepts of the idea: the attachment system is an inborn protective mechanism to keep the young close to those who care for them. It persists through adulthood, shaping various social relationships, including those with significant others as well as with such people as work supervisors and neighbors. According to one psychologist, adult attachment styles result from the fit between people's models of themselves and their models of others. People who feel generally positive about themselves and other people are described as having a secure attachment style. Those who have a negative, insecure sense of their own worth and value compared to their positive, idealistic view of others generally feel preoccupied and worried about whether they are truly liked and accepted by others. That same negative sense of the self, combined with a view of others as untrustworthy and unreliable, produces a fearful attachment style. But, when people have that negative view of others, combined with self-confidence and the belief that only the self can be counted on, they are dismissive of other people. An easy way to understand these four attachment styles can be seen in four quadrants (adapted from Bartholomew 1990, 163):

Model of self

	Positive	Negative
Positive	SECURE	PREOCCUPIED
Negative	DISMISSING	FEARFUL

Model of others

Developmental psychologists study attachment. Psychoanalysts theorize about object relations (e.g., Greenberg and Mitchell 1983). Social psychologists argue for the basic human need for belonging (e.g., Baumeister and Leary 1995). Neuroscientists observe parts of the brain that signal the distress of social isolation (e.g., Eisenberger and Lieberman 2004).[5] Philosophers reflect on the meaning of "persons in relation" (Macmurray 1961). We could add many other examples, but these few illustrate the convergence occurring today on the core idea of relationality. As the twentieth century drew to a close, scholarship in the sciences and humanities was declaring that this fundamental aspect of being human had gone missing, particularly in Western cultures, which embraced individualism, autonomy, and the rational mind.

All this talk of relationality, however, poses a challenge for those of us who care about persons who are living with dementia. Why are so many of them isolated from friends, family members, and the wider community?

Malignant Social Psychology and Dementia

Regardless of whether there are plaques and tangles accumulating in the brain and producing what we call Alzheimer's disease, and regardless of whether the brain shows signs of strokes or Lewy bodies or deterioration of the frontal lobes, the person experiencing these brain changes represents a complex history of social relationships implanted in body and mind from the earliest days of existence. Even before birth, the need to be in relation to others was woven into the genetic instructions that formed the nervous system. For persons who have dementia—including those living in the final days without language and little consciousness—relationships still matter, and gentle, loving touch can communicate human connectedness just as it did in infancy.[6] Remember the monkeys who were not touched by another monkey but desperately clung to their cloth mothers, and the babies who died when they had no one to cuddle and comfort them? How many people in nursing homes ever get a hug, much less the opportunity to curl up next to another human being who loves them?

Why is it so hard to understand that persons who have dementia need meaningful connections with other human beings? Why do so many people persist in thinking that the person who has dementia is "just an empty shell"? Tom Kitwood argued that we fail to see personhood in dementia because dementia has been constructed according to a medical model of limits and losses, creating what Stephen Sabat called a "defectological" (2001, 92) image, which reveals only what a person can no longer do. Kitwood, who died suddenly in 1998 at age 61, contradicted this image in his legacy of research, writing, and leadership in the world of dementia care, a legacy that has given hope to persons with the diagnosis and those who care for them. Hope is located not in the expectation of a medical miracle to eliminate symptoms of dementia but in positive relationships that affirm personhood at all points in the dementia journey. Hope lies in the elimination of what Kitwood called "malignant social psychology" (1997, 45).

We need to pause and think more deeply about this idea of malignant social psychology, for all of us have the potential to slip into social behaviors that malign the personhood of others. Kitwood said this is "part of our cultural inheritance" (1997, 46). We demonstrate malignant social psychology intentionally or inadvertently to family members, friends, colleagues, and strangers of all ages and mental capacities when we

- Deceive others in order to manipulate them
- Disempower people by not allowing them to do what they are still capable of doing
- Act in a patronizing, infantilizing way
- Intimidate others, making them fear our power and authority
- Apply dehumanizing labels
- Stigmatize others, treating them as if they are not fully human
- Outpace people who are slower than we are in behavior or verbal comprehension
- Invalidate others' experiences
- Exclude people physically or psychologically
- Treat a person as if he or she is an object to be moved about or "parked" in place
- Ignore people by "talking over their heads"
- Deny others the opportunity to make choices
- Blame people for things they cannot control
- "Elbow into" a person's activity, thus disrupting it

- Tease or make fun of another person
- Disparage a person as being incompetent

These behaviors produce "excess disability" (Brody et al. 1971) not only in persons who have dementia but also in persons who have other forms of disability, as well as in persons who give care.

Excess disability occurs when an individual's ability to function is impaired, not just by physical or mental problems,[7] but by other people's attitudes about their condition. We create excess disability when we shout at blind people (assuming for some reason that their hearing is also impaired) and when we treat a person who is living with dementia as if he or she is completely unaware of our presence. It is challenging enough to live with dementia—as the person with the diagnosis and as the person who gives care—without the additional burden of others who assume that you are no longer a person or that you are wasting your time in caregiving.

A good example of excess disability appeared in a story told by Richard and Bernice Lazarus in *Coping with Aging* (2006). The Lazaruses wrote this book when they were in their eighties and living at Rossmoor, a large adult community in northern California. There they had the opportunity to observe closely the ways excess disability was created and maintained, not by young people enchanted by their own youth, but by older people themselves. Dorothy and Gardner were living with Gardner's diagnosis of Alzheimer's disease. His symptoms began when he was about 65, just after they had moved to Rossmoor. The Lazaruses described how Gardner's increasing confusion coexisted with his determination to remain socially engaged. He grew agitated when he had trouble communicating, and more agitated when he realized that others had no patience with his troubles. "Gardner had become a nuisance and was making people uncomfortable. They began to avoid him, which only made him try harder. His actions conveyed the pathos of a vague understanding about what was happening to him and a desperate attempt to cover it up" (125).

Excess disability afflicted Gardner and also affected Dorothy. Although she was dedicated to looking after Gardner's needs and was doing a fine job, her friends increasingly urged her to "put him in a nursing home." This, of course, made her doubt her decision to care for her husband. She learned as much as she could about Alzheimer's disease, as well as about the disturbing emotions she shared with other care partners.[8] It did not help that some of her friends continued to "tell her to write Gardner off emotionally and attend to her own needs" (2006, 128). In contrast, a few of her friends seemed intuitively to understand the problem of excess disability. "They accepted Garner without complaint, despite his irrational behavior, and they tried to understand how Dorothy must be feeling. Some were helpful simply because they listened and did not prescribe. They made it clear by their loyalty and thoughtfulness that they cared and would not be judgmental. . . . Still others showed little patience for her plight and soon disappeared from sight" (129).

We have heard many similar stories about social malignancy and excess disability. For example, a chaplain told of a visit from a man who wished to talk with her about his difficult interactions with his wife. After he had been diagnosed with Alzheimer's disease, his wife responded by trying to take control of all aspects of his life. It seemed he could no longer make any decisions on his own. Even though he understood her behavior as a reflection of her own anxiety about his condition, this treatment was making him angry and frustrated. He was afraid he would blow up at her and that his anger would be attributed to "the disease" and not to his feeling that his very selfhood was being suffocated by his wife's behavior. He came to see a chaplain about this problem because he experienced it as a spiritual issue. He viewed his spirituality as being the ground of his relationships.

It may have struck some readers in thinking about Kitwood's work that there is a deep moral and even spiritual tone running through it. Indeed, Kitwood acknowledged this repeatedly, saying that how we view the personhood of those who have dementia implies a moral obligation to eliminate the malignant social psychology. Moreover, he stated that this view of personhood requires a psychology that focuses on "experience, action, and spirituality" (1997, 55).

Kitwood's psychological approach to dementia was richly broad and integrative, ranging across levels of analysis from the neurological to the spiritual. This may sound like a rather tall order, out of synch with the materialism of some psychological thinking. However, if we consider spirituality to be an expression of the human need for meaning and self-transcendence, and if we accept that all experience and action (include our striving for meaning and self-transcendence) is expressed through the nervous system and leaves an imprint on it, then it is not so hard to see how Kitwood might make this claim. In this passage, one can observe how Kitwood set this integrative approach within a lifespan view of human life that sees the older person as bearing a personal history that has shaped consciousness:

> As an infant responds to others, processes that are at first interpersonal become
> "internalized"—part of the individual psyche. At the same time the central ner-

vous system is growing and maturing, holding the fruit of experience in place. In dementia many aspects of the psyche that had for a long time, been individual and "internal," are again made over to the interpersonal milieu. Memory may have faded, but something of the past is known; identity remains intact, because others hold it in place; thoughts may have disappeared, but there are still interpersonal processes; feelings are expressed and meet a validating response; and if there is a spirituality, it will most likely be of the kind that Buber describes, where the divine is encountered in the depth of I-Thou relating. (1997, 69)

Perhaps it was not so strange for Kitwood the psychologist to have integrated a spiritual perspective into his views on personhood, dementia, and dementia care. He was an ordained Anglican priest and served as a school chaplain before his life took a turn toward psychology and work with persons who have dementia.

Today, interest in spirituality and dementia is growing both within and outside of traditional religious environments.[9] We explore this topic in greater depth in later chapters, but for now, we wade ever so lightly into theology, a place Kitwood invited us to explore through his embrace of Buber's work and its description of the essence of the I-Thou meeting as grace: a gift we do not seek but which is freely offered by a loving other, or Other. In addition, Kitwood's work invites theological reflection because in the years since his death in 1998, theological scholarship about disability has proliferated.[10] Kitwood insisted that "dementing illnesses should be seen, primarily, as forms of disability" (1997, 136), an idea that is just beginning to gain some traction in the dementia-care community.

Theological Perspectives on Disability

Theologian and ethicist Stanley Hauerwas argues that our deepest fears grow from those conditions that most threaten our fundamental sense of identity as a self. In the time of Jesus, prevailing cultural and religious assumptions held that corporal bodies constituted the self, and therefore the most dreaded disease was leprosy, which represented losing one's self as the physical body become more disfigured.

Because the Jewish and Christian traditions have long associated selfhood with the *imago Dei*—the conviction that humans are uniquely created in the image of God—the loss of corporal wholeness (through leprosy, castration, amputation, etc.) was believed to damage the divine image in which we are created.

Lepers were therefore barred from entering the sacred temple, effectively deny-ing them access to the transcendent realm. Purity laws also demanded that lep-ers be prohibited from physical contact with other persons and removed from their normal role in the web of relationships that constitute community. Lep-rosy thus cost its victim relationship with self, relationship with the divine, and relationship with the community. Jesus' first response to lepers, Hauerwas notes, was to touch them, and through that touch, to offer the healing knowledge that the leper remained a person—a self valued by God and capable of continu-ing relationship with fellow human beings.

In the constructs of modernity, cultural and religious assumptions about the nature of the self have moved from corporality to cognition, from body to mind. The *imago Dei* is now commonly associated with such terms as *intelligence, auto-nomy,* and *independence.* Our deepest fears are therefore less associated with physical well-being than with cognitive well-being; they are centered on those conditions that threaten this new understanding of self, namely, Alzheimer's and other forms of dementia. For many, Alzheimer's represents the loss of self-hood, and people moving into dementia often say "I am losing myself, one piece of my mind (memory) at a time."

Like leprosy in a different era, dementia threatens the ability to maintain a relationship with the divine and to sustain social roles within community.[11] Par-ticularly in religious traditions that emphasize sermons or homilies, it is often assumed that a family member who has dementia should no longer participate in corporate worship because "he doesn't get anything out of it." Persons on the dementia road are often effectively pronounced "unclean" and hidden away as if contagious, living in a world populated solely by family members and paid care-givers rather than friends and community. Long-time companions on life's jour-ney may distance themselves from the friend who has Alzheimer's disease, jus-tifying this distance with words like "He has already left us" or "I want to remember her as she was." Hauerwas points back to Jesus touching the lepers, suggesting that the first response to a friend who has Alzheimer's should be to touch him or her.[12]

In the last thirty years, a significant literature on the theology of disability has developed, beginning with the pioneering essays on intellectual disabilities (for-merly called mental retardation) authored by Hauerwas (1986).[13] Among other persons who have made significant contributions to this conversation are Jean Vanier and Henri Nouwen, of the L'Arche network of communities, John Swin-ton, Hans Reinders, and Thomas Reynolds. Although their perspectives range widely, a common thread linking their diverse works is the conviction that persons living with disabilities confront us with the inadequacy of existing cultural and religious understandings of personhood and the *imago Dei*. Persons who are traveling the dementia road raise the same fundamental challenges and point the way to similar new understandings of what constitutes personhood and the *imago Dei*, so it is important to review the challenges this literature raises and the new understandings to which it points.

The conviction that human beings stand above and apart from the rest of natural creation by virtue of their intellect has been broadly accepted by both religious and nonreligious people. From Psalm 8 ("You have made them a little lower than God, and crowned them with glory and honor") to Shakespeare ("What a piece of work is a man, how noble in reason, how infinite in faculties, in form and moving how express and admirable, in action how like an angel, in apprehension how like a god!"),[14] there is longstanding consensus that the human being, "the reasoning animal," represents the crowning achievement of the Almighty.

This persistent conviction (or remarkable hubris) has been upheld by writings in religious anthropology that have sought to enumerate the intrinsic traits and abilities unique to human beings that affirm their privileged place within the created order: abstract thought, use of tools, language, altruism, and a host of others. One by one the majority of these "unique" traits has fallen to empirical research, and only a few stones remain in the shrinking foundation of presumed human uniqueness. Yet the belief that selfhood and the *imago Dei* are rooted in human intellect remains as persistent today as it did in the era of foundational Christian theologians such as Augustine ("by giving him a rational soul, which raises him above the beasts in the field")[15] and Aquinas ("only in a rational creature do you find a resemblance to God in a manner of an image").[16]

But if intellect alone defines the *imago Dei*, it would seem to follow that the brightest person among us would be the most "godly," apart from his or her moral character or compassion for others. As Martin Luther grumbled, "if these powers alone are the image of God it follows that Satan was created according to the image of God, since he surely has these natural endowments . . . to a far higher degree than we have them."[17] Just as critically, defining the *imago Dei* through reason and intellect alone would seem to suggest that persons born with profound cognitive disability were not fully created in the divine image and that those who lose cognitive ability through accident or disease have had the divine image stripped from them.

The Cult of Normalcy

Theologian Thomas Reynolds (himself the father of a multiply disabled child) argues that a community's perception of disability "is the inverse projection of its own framework of normalcy" (2008, 33). That is to say, without a consensus on what constitutes "normal" for personhood, we cannot gauge which persons fall outside such norms because of perceived physical or cognitive limitations. We tend to consider those so identified as victims to be pitied and to sympathize with their suffering (whether or not the persons themselves are experiencing pain, discomfort, or unhappiness).

Reynolds traces the ways in which disability has been theologically denigrated or trivialized by exploring Hebrew and Christian scriptures that have been interpreted to portray disability as divine punishment for disobedience,[18] as an expression of inadequate faith,[19] or as a special gift granted to "virtuous sufferers" whose condition provides spiritual depth (as in Paul's mysterious "thorn in the flesh") or brings particular blessings to the community (too often used sentimentally to describe a child who has Down syndrome as "a special blessing from God"). Reynolds points out that other texts clearly state that suffering, disease, and disability are neither willed nor caused by God,[20] and they lift up a broader vision of spiritual community defined by love and inclusion.[21]

Drawing from the work of Erving Goffman on stigma and anthropologist Mary Douglas on taboo, Reynolds traces what he terms "the cult of normalcy" from multiple sources,[22] including religious paradigms that divided the created order into the acceptable and unacceptable, the holy and the abominable. Reynolds quotes Mary Douglas on the priestly dietary restrictions of ancient Israel: "In the firmament two-legged fowls fly with wings. In the water scaly fish swim with fins. On the earth four-legged animals hop, jump or walk. Any class of creatures which is not equipped for the right kind of locomotion in its element is contrary to holiness. Contact with it disqualifies a person from approaching the Temple. Thus anything in the water which has not fins and scales is unclean (Lev. 11:10–12)" (Douglas 1966, quoted in Reynolds 2008, 65).

Once such distinctions between the normal and the abnormal became established, they were easily extended to gender, class, race, ethnicity, sexual orientation, and health. In determining who was normal and who was not, we came to regard those labeled "abnormal" as persons to be shunned, pitied, cured, or "fixed." Modernity brought us the bell curve, where the person who is normal occupies the center of the curve and those who fail to conform to that norm are progressively marginalized by being pushed to the outer edges. The risks of such a model are well illustrated by Goffman's (1963) sarcastic description of the prototypical male figure in North American culture: "a young, married, white, urban, northern, heterosexual Protestant father of college education, fully employed, of good complexion, weight, and height, and a recent record in sports" (128). Too often our conception of the normal is an idealized, unattainable image by which we view persons with physical or cognitive disabilities as damaged or deficient. Reynolds (2008) sees this dynamic as particularly dangerous when applied by "the medical model and its desire to cure the 'deficiencies' of the disabled body. Normalcy is legitimated in terms of its contrast, the abnormal, which is invested with all kinds of negative connotations, perhaps even to the point of being evil" (62).

Reynolds (2008) aptly captures the consensus conception of what constitutes personhood in liberal Enlightenment understanding: "an autonomous and self-determining individual capable of entering into social collaboration on the basis of rational self-interest. Reason is that which enables us to govern our own lives in the private sphere, and reach agreement with others in the public sphere. And its benchmark is autonomy" (80).

This is less a definition than an ideology. It privileges the mind at the expense of the body and the individual at the expense of the community. It serves the interests of a materialistic culture, in which a person's worth is measured in terms of productivity, accumulation of wealth, and consumption of goods. In such a culture, persons are understood to be individuals in competition with one another to attain scarce resources rather than as mutually dependent participants in the task of building a common community where all persons can flourish. Those with disabilities or those who travel the dementia road are viewed as "damaged goods," no longer able to produce or compete. The aging of the American population is framed in terms of the economic burden it will lay on individual taxpayers, using the alarmist language of "apocalyptic demography" (Moody 2002, 45; see also Robertson 1990). Disability and dementia become the problem of individuals and their families rather than a shared experience within the human community in which all participate. In both cultural and religious terms, this is a reductionist understanding of personhood that isolates persons from one another and alienates them from their place within the created order. Persons living with disability or dementia challenge us to rethink what it is to be a person created in the divine image and to build new structures of community in which people think of one another as friends and neighbors rather than as competitors.

Western society has been profoundly shaped by the myths of the rugged individual and the self-made man or woman who has worked his or her way to the top by virtue of intellect, will, and disciplined effort. If such images are permitted to define normal human experience and reside at the top of the bell curve defining personhood, then not just the disabled but the great majority of human beings fail to meet the standards of normalcy and full personhood. If we return to the notion with which we began—that we dread most that which threatens our sense of self—we should ask what it is that the person with profound disability or who travels the dementia road says about us that we do not wish to see or hear. Reynolds' answer is that they present us with the truth that "we are incomplete, vulnerable, and need others to become complete" (2008, 106).

Selfhood and Relationality

We are vulnerable because suffering is a necessary and unavoidable part of human experience. We suffer physical injuries and emotional wounds, disappointments, and losses. We suffer because of illness or natural disaster. We suffer setbacks in our dreams and projects. We suffer from the effects of violence and war. Because we are human, we suffer. As Hauerwas (1986) notes, "We suffer because we are incomplete beings who depend upon one another for our existence. Indeed, the matter can be put more strongly, since we depend upon others not only for our survival but also for our identity. Suffering is built into our condition because it is literally true that we exist only to the extent that we sustain, or 'suffer,' the existence of others" (169).

We have seen that much of the effort to define selfhood and the *imago Dei* has focused on intrinsic traits or abilities assumed to be unique to human beings—corporeal form, intellect, autonomy, and so on. But while it may be legitimate to employ such intrinsic traits and abilities to define humans as distinct from other living creatures, what makes us human does not necessarily make us a "self" created in the image of the divine. Rather, it is our extrinsic relationships with other persons that confer on us our identity as a "self," and it is the loving relationship that God maintains with us that constitutes the *imago Dei*—we are creatures in God's image only because God chooses to be in relationship with us. Because God's love is unconditional, this relationship cannot be broken by human limitations—the disabled person or the person traveling the dementia road is no less valued or loved by God, nor is he or she less capable of sharing joyous, sustaining relationship with other persons. If our relationships are, as Reynolds and others insist, what define us as a person, then all of us are dependent on others to grant us the gift of selfhood.

Theologian Karl Barth tied the concept of "relationship" to that of "freedom." God created men and women in the image of God's own freedom, and it is in this freedom that we most resemble God. But this freedom is not modernity's "freedom from" expressed in the language of personal rights ("nobody can tell me what to do"). Rather it is a "freedom for," above all the freedom to engage in committed relationships with others.

Such freedom forms and maintains relationships not for personal gain but because it is through relationships that genuine freedom is expressed. A sentimental cliché has it that "God made men and women because God was lonely and needed someone to talk to." But a lonely God who needs us for companionship would not be a god at all. When God provided Moses a name by which God could be called, it was an affirmation that God chooses to be in relationship with human beings. The very name that was given—*Yahweh,* which defies tidy translation into English but can be loosely rendered as "I am what I am"—made it clear that God is completely Other and does not require relationship with human beings to meet God's own needs. A pastor who was challenged to summarize the entire Bible in a single sentence made this noble effort: "I am God and you are not!"

The Christian doctrine of the Trinity likewise speaks of God's self-sufficiency, for God is understood to be in perfect, continuous relationship within God's own being. But God's internal relationship does not stand apart from God's external relationship with men and women. Meister Eckhart, the thirteenth-century mystic, expressed the connection between God's internal and external relationships in this manner, as translated by Raymond Blakney: "When God laughs at the soul and the soul laughs back at God, the persons of the Trinity are begotten. To speak in hyperbole, when the Father laughs to the Son and the Son laughs back to the Father, that laughter gives pleasure, that pleasure gives joy, that joy gives love, and love gives the persons [of the Trinity] of which the Holy Spirit is one" (Blakney 1941, 245).

Eckhart gives poetic expression to a web of human/divine relationship that is as mysterious as it is wondrous. Relationships that give expression to true freedom—whether within God's own being, between God and human beings, or between persons—are marked by pleasure, joy, and love. The presence or absence of intrinsic qualities such as intellect or autonomy has no bearing on the ability to be in a relationship where joy and love are given and received.

Hans Reinders (2008) explains how Barth found the interconnectedness of freedom, creation, and relationship expressed in the Trinity: "In Barth's terminology, God's act of freedom exists in the addressing, the being addressed, and the address itself. It is the loving Father who is addressing, it is the beloved Son who is being addressed, and it is the Spirit of love that is the address passing between them. . . . Therefore, in terms of the 'I-Thou' language that Barth prefers at this point, God's addressing 'I' relates to the divine 'Thou' that is thus being addressed . . . and thus human creatures relate to one another as 'I' and 'Thou' " (239).

The language of "I-Thou" employed by Barth (and also by Tom Kitwood) is most often associated with philosopher Martin Buber (1970), who distinguished between "I-Thou" and "I-it" relationships. In the former, we encounter other persons in the awareness that the one with whom we relate is not an "object" we can control or manipulate. The "Thou" we address carries within himself or herself a unity of being that cannot be reduced to specific qualities that can be enumerated, weighed, or measured. We can never fully know or comprehend the person we address as "Thou." We can only honor and enjoy the one we call "Thou."

Such a relationship is distinct from the "I-it" relationship we have with an inanimate object, a "thing" that can be used for whatever purpose we wish. Unfortunately, many human relationships fall into the second category, in which one person treats another as an object that can be moved like a piece on a chessboard. We place our dinner order with the waiter or wait impatiently while the woman at the counter rings up our groceries, barely aware that we are in the presence of a fellow human being. A physician sees a patient as a set of symptoms to be evaluated as quickly as possible rather than as a whole being to be cherished.

In "I-it" relationships, the world is populated by knowable objects we are free to use, including fellow human beings. In "I-Thou" relationships there is always an element of sacred mystery: we share in a common reality in which each of us can know and be known but never fully understood. For Buber, God is the "divine Thou" who sustains the "I-Thou" relationship eternally. Buber was speaking out of his Jewish faith, yet there are significant similarities between his "I-Thou" and the descriptions Eckhart and Barth offer of Christianity's Triune God, whose internal relationship is an eternal "I-Thou," as is God's relationship with human beings. In relating to one another as "I-Thou," we bring an element of transcendent mystery to our understanding of what it is to be a self.

If we understand each person, no matter what his or her condition or circumstances may be, as a "Thou"—a unified whole who cannot be reduced to specific traits, abilities, or symptoms and who we are not free to use for our own purposes—we must reject the claims of the cult of normalcy that count some people as limited or defective in ways that make them something less than fully a person. Each human life begins in vulnerability and dependence on others, conditions that continue to define us each day that we live (whether we care to admit it or not). Sometimes our vulnerability and dependence on others will become obvious—when we have suffered an accident or major illness or lost a cherished companion to death—but even when it is not obvious it remains true. We may succeed, at least for a period of time, in convincing ourselves of the myth that we are autonomous and independent, but inevitably we must rely on others for everything that makes life rich and good.

In our relationships, we learn both the joy of giving and the joy of receiving; only through interactions with other persons can we be fully formed as persons. Evolutionary biologists and psychologists assert that as vulnerable, dependent creatures we are hard-wired to be in relationship with other persons. Theologians are more likely to say that we were created to be in committed, sustaining friendships with one another.

CHAPTER FOUR

What Is Friendship?

What is a friend? A teen might answer, "My friends are the people I like to hang out with." Adults may speak of the people who share their tastes and interests. Sometimes we speak of friends in terms of the settings in which we interact: our "work friends" or our "friends at the lake." In the new world of social networking, people speak of their "Facebook friends" or "Twitter friends." A common thread is a sense of connectedness—a network of persons whom we like and enjoy (and who, we hope, like and enjoy us in return).

Probe a bit deeper and people may speak of true friends as "the folks who will be there for me when I need them." We move beyond casual connection to loyalty and commitment because our lives have become intertwined in a manner that permits friends to have meaningful expectations of one another.

In this chapter, we explore friendship from the perspectives of the social sciences and one particular philosopher: Aristotle. First, we note the challenges gerontologists have encountered in trying to understand friendship, a relationship that "persons on the street" have little trouble describing but which causes social scientists all kinds of difficulties when they try to put it under their lens and study it. One of their research challenges is that friendships exist in time, and personal choices and life circumstances sometimes cause disruptions in friendships.

For older people, of course, the greatest and most painful disruption of friendship is the final one, when the friend dies. Visit any assisted-living residence or nursing home and you will find very old people who will tell you that *everyone* they were ever close to—family members and friends—is gone. Because human beings are fundamentally relational, as we explained in the last chapter, many of these elders form new friendships with fellow residents. They will tell you that these friendships are not the same as the ones with persons they had known for so many years; some will also say that they are reluctant to become close to others because they know that death haunts even the cheeriest and most progressive place where old people live. Nevertheless, spend a little time there, and you will see much evidence of people caring for one another. They check on one another's welfare, greet one another in the hallways, share meals and activities, worry when someone's health declines, argue about things, and joke and laugh together.

In "congregate living facilities" (to use terminology gerontologists sometimes employ), with a variety of types of service, ranging from very little for the so-called independent residents to skilled-nursing care and memory care, dementia can be a major challenge to social networks. The "well elderly" often actively avoid contact with those who have severe memory loss for a variety of reasons: not wanting to be reminded of their own potential for forgetfulness or simply not knowing how to interact with people who are living with dementia. On the other hand, in such settings one can also observe persons who have advanced dementia experiencing meaningful and loving friendships. Here are two stories that illustrate just a few of the many possible expressions and forms of friendship to be found today in residences for older people.

Louise and her husband, Tom, have lived at the Harbor, a continuum-of-care retirement community for about one year. A retired nurse, she has been diagnosed with early stage dementia, although one might not know that on first meeting her. She and Tom feel strongly about reaching out to other people. For example, Louise describes how they make a point of inviting "new people" to sit at their table in the dining room. Both are acutely aware of the dynamics of social networks at the Harbor, especially the "clique-ish-ness" of some of the residents, who are friendly to only a select few. Louise admits, however, that despite the strong value she places on friendliness, she is not sure how to deal with people who are more confused than she. This comes up repeatedly in her bridge group. She has been an avid bridge player her whole life. The game gives her great pleasure, but she is increasingly concerned about what she should do about friends who are progressing quickly with memory loss, so much so that the shared activity they have all enjoyed for so many years is affected.

Rosie and Bess lived in a memory care unit at the Greens. Rosie had been there for several years when Bess arrived. Both had such severe dementia that they rarely spoke. When they did speak, no one could understand what they were trying to say. Nevertheless, staff members noticed that the two women seemed to have formed an important friendship around their both being devoutly Catholic. In this facility, made up of small households of about eleven persons, each resident has a private room, and the families of Rosie and Bess had decorated their rooms with many symbols of their faith. Rosie and Bess pointed to these symbols in one another's rooms; they sat next to each other at the weekly gatherings for praying the rosary. On some level, they appeared to know that the other was what young people today call a soul mate. About six months after her arrival at the Greens, Bess died. That day, her daughter sat weeping in the commons area of the household. No one knows exactly how Rosie knew about Bess's death, because no one had yet had a chance to talk with the residents, but Rosie approached Bess's daughter and said, "I'm sorry for your loss. She was my friend."

Many factors determine who remains a friend over time and who becomes a friend late in life. Because dementia is by definition the experience of progressive forgetfulness, by necessity it brings change over time to the relationship regardless of whether the friendship has spanned many decades or less than a year. Because this book is addressed primarily to persons who have not given much thought to what will happen to their own friendships when forgetfulness increases, most of the examples in this chapter describe relationships more like the ones Louise is attempting to negotiate and less like the friendship of Rosie and Bess. Nevertheless, it is important to keep Rosie and Bess in mind as we examine gerontologists' studies of late-life friendships and Aristotle's ideas about virtuous friends. As we will see, Rosie and Bess shared a virtuous friendship.

Friendship Viewed through the Lens of Gerontology

Gerontologists usually describe their work as addressing aging as a process, old age as a period in the life course, and older adults' individual characteristics and situational circumstances. Large national gatherings of these people who spend much of their time thinking about aging, old age, and older adults can be dizzying affairs. Researchers and practitioners scurry from one conference session to another, occasionally plop down in lobby chairs to chat with colleagues seen but once a year, wave to one another on escalators, and roam through large rooms (usually several floors underground) where purveyors of books and programs and apparatus for elders display their wares. A talk about the role of the arts in dementia care might take place in a hotel meeting room next to one where a physician is describing the latest approach to clinical care for elder athletes. Down the hall, someone might be showing PowerPoint slides of brain scans, while on another floor of the conference site, a social worker describes new programs at meal sites for low-income elders. Sometimes the "splitting" of categories of aging that we described in the Introduction is painfully felt at these conferences. The presentations on various components of living well in old age[1]— sometimes described as attributes of "successful aging"—can seem separate from those addressing the lives of persons with progressive memory loss.

The plethora of professional identities and topics addressed at gatherings of gerontologists can be inspiring and exhausting at the same time. Not only do gerontologists come from an enormous array of disciplinary homes,[2] but they also have different kinds of professional identities. One way of simplifying this is to think of the three-legged stool, not of income sources for older adults (Social Security, pensions, personal savings) but of research, practice, and public policy. All three are necessary to meet gerontology's goal of late-life well-being, which itself can be described as reflecting a complex intersection of environmental, financial, physical, psychological, social, and spiritual characteristics. All this is to say that when gerontologists turn their attention to a phenomenon like friendship, they approach it from a number of disciplinary and professional "standing grounds."[3]

Scanning the literature on friendship, one quickly discovers that sociologists have been thinking about it for a much longer time than psychologists (although as we will see later in this chapter, no one can beat the philosophers, going back to Aristotle). Sociologists usually examine the external structures of life, such as social roles, which affect the formation and endurance of friendship. As roles change, friendships may change. For example, people form friendships at work, but if they relocate after retiring and do not remain in contact with friends from work, the connections may be lost. Sociologists also attend to the influence of individual-difference markers on friendship, such as a person's age, gender, race, or ethnic heritage. Psychologists tend to be more interested in what individuals bring to the relationship in terms of personality characteristics that affect comfort with emotional closeness. In gerontology, the lines between these two disciplines become blurred, for persons from both disciplines agree on the importance of accounting for the dynamic interaction between psychological dispositions and social structures that affects how people behave with friends, how they think about friendship, and how they feel about individual friends and friendship in general. Moreover, because gerontologists are acutely aware of heterogeneity among older people, they situate their work on friendship within social, cultural, and historical contexts.[4]

One well-known friendship researcher boldly stated that in the social sciences (where psychology and sociology are usually categorized), the people studying aging, old age, and older people—in other words, the gerontologists—have focused the most attention on friendship (Adams 1997).[5] However, gerontologists have not always agreed with one another's views on older people's social relationships. This was especially true through the 1960s, as gerontologists argued over whether older people preferred staying just as socially active as they had been earlier in their lives or whether they chose to disengage from social relationships as they withdrew from various role responsibilities and turned inward to tap their own resources for well-being. The so-called activity theorists produced research showing that older adults maintained contacts with friendship networks and found new friends when old friendships were severed due to retirement, relocation, or death. On the disengagement side of the argument, some gerontologists highlighted the inward turn taken by some older people as they shed the responsibilities and roles that had occupied their attention earlier in adulthood.[6] Whether this inward turn necessarily implied a turn away from friends became a point of contention. Some in this argument noted that because older people were losing friends to death and frailty, perhaps they had no choice but to disengage in order to protect themselves from the pain of accumulating loss. Others saw disengagement as being less a choice than a condition forced on older people because of social prejudices against the old.

Finally, as often happens when researchers stake their claims on one side or another of a controversy over how human beings live, by the mid-1970s, most gerontologists had concluded that "it all depends" is the best answer to the question about how older people structure their social lives. People vary in their attitudes about friendship, friendship skills, and need for friends. Life circumstances affect friendship, too. Sometimes by choice and sometimes by chance, social relationships can change as people age.

Robert Atchley, a widely respected social gerontologist (meaning that his disciplinary roots lie in sociology), provided a helpful way of thinking about this by articulating a "continuity theory" of aging (1989, 1999). Longitudinal data that he collected for many years from a group of individuals aging in Ohio showed that what older adults most wanted was continuity in their lives. In other words, those who had many close friendships through middle adulthood usually wanted to stay socially active, while those who had always had fewer close friends continued to value those relationships while not actively seeking new friends. Atchley wrote that aging persons strive to maintain both an internal sense of continuity, experienced as an ongoing sense of selfhood and identity, as well as an external continuity of environments and connections with familiar persons.

The dialectic between internal and external experience is complex and dynamic, for gerontologists must always account for the passage of time.[7] This is why longitudinal studies like Atchley's are considered the "gold standard" for research on aging: they allow researchers to follow the same group of individuals over many years, observing how people affect their environments and how environments (which include other human beings) affect people. As time passes, our bodies undergo both predictable and unpredictable changes. Changes occur in what we know about our lives and the world and how we interpret that knowledge. Our emotional lives unfold over time, in terms of both the internal process of regulation of our emotional responses and the external events that elicit those responses. Our needs and desires can change, and even as these cognitive, affective, and motivational developments are occurring, the outer world is also changing. Our friends are growing older even as we ourselves are aging. As the country rock group Son Volt puts it in their song "Tear-Stained Eye," we are on a road together, experiencing the "traveling hands of time."

One of the most powerful metaphors in gerontology expressing the effects of the passage of time on social relationships appeared in an edited volume in 1980. In their chapter, Robert Kahn and Toni Antonucci (1980) gave students of aging the image of the social convoy.

During the gasoline crisis of 1973–74, Americans became aware of convoys because convoys of truckers were moving slowly along interstate highways protesting fuel prices and rationing. Imagine a bird's-eye view of a typical interstate highway in ordinary times (that is, when you do not have more than forty trucks deliberately traveling slowly together). Gazing down on three lanes heading west, you might see nine or ten 18-wheel behemoths all bunched up together. Sometimes one pulls ahead, then drops back, and another takes the lead. Occasionally, a truck exits, perhaps heading north, never to join that particular convoy again. But, sometimes, the exit is only for a pit stop, just a bit of time apart from the convoy. A few of the trucks tend to stay close together, while the others move along the periphery of the convoy. Perhaps the drivers of the ones traveling closer together have become friends over the years of driving back and forth across America, whereas the others are more distant acquaintances, to be greeted with a nod at rest stops. And speaking of rest stops, and extending the metaphor a bit further, we can picture the convoy as including not just the truckers driving along the interstate but also the people they regularly meet along the way who provide essential services to keep the trucks moving and the drivers fed.

Now imagine a group a friends who met during their college years. They spent three or four years "hanging out" together; as a convoy they traveled the hands of time together for a while. But then jobs and families and other adult obligations took them in different directions. A few may have stayed in close contact, but connections with others were severed forever, whether purposefully or because of the accumulation of differing life priorities. Later, sometimes many years later, they might meet up again and reconnect in a relationship that endures. Or, they might simply get together for a drink when by chance they happen to be in the same city and then connect no more.

Obviously, this convoy metaphor looks very different for family members, for regardless of whether there is emotional closeness, the familial relationship continues over time. My cousin is always my cousin, even though I may not have seen him for thirty years and feel no emotional connection to him. We are both aging. Someday he may pop up on my Facebook site and a relationship may be renewed—or not.

Kahn and Antonucci (1980) illustrated the changing composition of social convoys with two different concentric circles indicating the closeness and density of relationships for a woman imagined at age 35 and again at age 75. The younger woman has her parents, husband, sister, and several friends in the ring closest to her; moving out from that ring, in the next one are several other siblings, neighbors, and some college friends. In the furthest ring (but still a part of the convoy) are her husband's friends, more neighbors, co-workers, etc. In comparison, the older woman's concentric rings have far fewer people occupying them.

Kahn and Antonucci described the essence of the convoy as movement "though the life cycle surrounded by a set of other people to whom [we are] related by the giving and receiving of social support" (269). In their model, social support consists of transactions of "affect, affirmation, and aid" (267). We like, admire, respect, and even love persons in our convoy. We affirm them by letting them know that we appreciate and value the choices they make. We give aid in a host of different ways, ranging from material assistance to information to emotional comfort. The shrinking population of the concentric circles that occurs with aging does not necessarily have to reduce the level of affect, affirmation, and aid they receive, although that is certainly an outcome for many older people.

The twenty-first century world of social networking via Facebook, Twitter, MySpace, and other Websites has added a new element to the notion of the social convoy. Although these began as ways for young, technologically astute people to connect, baby boomers have joined these digital convoys in great numbers. The question of how friendship is initiated, supported, and perhaps broken in these digital realms remains for researchers to address. Moreover, because they are so new, we do not yet know whether people will eventually tire of the effort needed to maintain digital contacts or whether their friendships in cyberspace will grow stronger as the years pass.

Our focus in this book—dementia, friendship, and community—addresses the issue of what happens to the social convoy when one or more of its members begins to experience progressive forgetfulness. Family members usually remain constant in their loyalty and love (although we know that sometimes certain family members struggle to maintain relationships with loved ones who are living with dementia). But, in the realm of friendship, will persons diagnosed with memory loss exit the convoy forever or will others in the convoy without memory problems make accommodations and offer support for staying "on board?" Will they join other convoys, perhaps online, in the early stages of memory loss when they can gather in digital discussion forums, or will they connect in person through groups sponsored by organizations like the Alzheimer's Association? As the memory loss accumulates, will they be forced to join a convoy of the fading and dying, one in which the only persons in the social network of daily life are others with progressive forgetfulness or much younger persons paid to care for them? Is there any place for friendship in this scenario and if so, what forms will it take?

Researchers are only beginning to address these questions. One Dutch study observed older people over the course of six years (Aartsen et al. 2004). Some of them experienced cognitive decline, others experienced physical decline, and a small percentage (7%) experienced both. Progressive memory loss and confusion resulted in a greater shrinkage of the network of close social relationships than was true for persons with increasing physical difficulties. Even family members who had originally been a part of the convoy of elders with cognitive difficulties drifted away. This effect was stronger for persons who initially had a relatively large network, perhaps because when there were more family, friends, and neighbors, each thought the other would be giving more attention to the person with cognitive problems. Social psychologists call this the "free rider" effect, meaning that in larger networks, people are "inclined to minimize their investments in relationships and maximize the profits" (Aartsen et al. 2004, 263).

As we observed in the last chapter, dementia is a condition intimately connected to time. By its very nature, it progresses. Moreover, not only is the person who is living with dementia experiencing changes in cognitive function over time, but other changes are taking place as well. Hair gets grayer or sparser, skin continues to wrinkle, and chronic afflictions of aging like arthritis become more problematic. Other persons on the convoy, regardless of which of its "circles" they occupy, are also experiencing the "traveling hands of time" and trying to find a good fit between their inner, psychological resources and the outer aspects of their lives, which involve social relationships experienced in various physical environments. Thus, we see how challenging it is to add to this complex aging scenario a notion like friendship, with all its many forms and meanings. And, we have not even attempted to *define* friendship yet!

So What *Is* Friendship?

So far in this chapter, we have talked about the difficulties of studying friendship and aging because of the complexities of each, the varying "standing grounds" of gerontologists, and the complicating matter of time. However, we have avoided the definitional dilemma and now must face it directly. Even though it is easy to look up a word like *friendship* in the dictionary, when it comes to discussing types and ideals of friendship, one finds many different approaches and emphases.

Those folks attending the gerontology conferences described earlier—people who may or may not have friendship or even dementia "on their screens" as they think about aging, old age, and older persons—can be sorted into roughly four broad categories based on disciplinary and professional standing grounds: social scientists, who most often work in academic settings, where they conduct research and teach; professionals in fields like medicine and social work who teach, do research, or provide direct care for older people and their families; program and institutional administrators; and, finally, the people who often insultingly get grouped into the "other" or "miscellaneous" category—people whose work in the arts and humanities should play a vital role in any gerontological discussion but who often struggle to have their voices heard over the din of biomedical and social scientific research that quantifies human lives and experiences.

Each of these groups comprises persons with their own experiences of being and having friends. Additionally, their scholarly backgrounds and work roles influence their theoretical and empirical approaches to friendship in particular ways. As we will see shortly, the social scientists gather and sort observations, sometimes guided by models or theories, and sometimes not. Persons associated with medical fields view friendship through the lens of research on its contributions to health. Administrators must consider whether their programs and institutions provide support for friendship (because they have probably read the biomedical research on how having a close confidant predicts late-life physical and mental well-being). People working in the arts and humanities have the deepest and widest heritage of reflection on friendship to draw on, for friendship has been considered by poets, artists, philosophers, and others since the beginning of recorded history.

As we wade into this thicket of reflections on friendship, we have chosen to begin by considering one of the oldest approaches, one identified with the humanities: Aristotle's reflections on types of friendship and the characteristics of a "complete" friendship. Only after we consider that ancient but still compelling treatment of the ideals of friendship will we turn to the descriptive approaches of contemporary social scientists.

Aristotle Teaches Us about Friendship

In his *Nicomachean Ethics*,[8] Aristotle (383–322 BCE) established a framework that still informs our understanding of friendship. The Greek term for friendship—*philia*—is broader than its English counterpart, encompassing all familiar acquaintances, including family members and business associates. Given this wide range of relationships, Aristotle grouped them into three broad categories: friendships based on utility, friendships based on pleasure, and friendships based on virtue.

Friendships based on *utility* have the quality of a business transaction—what can this person offer to me and what must I give in return in order to receive it? It is worth noting, and perhaps lamenting, that many social friendships in our culture carry strong elements of the utilitarian. Our friends are the people who can advance our career, drive our children to daycare, or grant us entrée to a desired social circle. When such a friendship no longer serves our needs, it is easily abandoned. Aristotle termed utilitarian friendships incomplete because they are motivated by immediate needs and contingent on circumstances that can quickly change. Too easily, the person whose company we once enjoyed on a regular basis can become just another name on our holiday card list.

Aristotle also defined friendships based on *pleasure* as incomplete. These are the friendships celebrated in advertisements and popular television programs: friendships between persons who cheer for the same sports teams, purchase the same consumer goods, hold similar political views, and make jokes about the same popular culture references. Such homogeneous friendships carry an element of narcissism, as we seek the company of persons who affirm our tastes and make us feel interesting and valued. Our friends are the people who are "just like us."

In Aristotle's view, a friendship that is complete shares elements with incomplete friendships—that is, it includes mutual helpfulness and enjoyment—but its primary center is in *virtue*: true friends support one another in the effort to live good and ethical lives. Aristotle described five features of such a friendship:

We wish good for our friends and seek to do good on their behalf;

We want our friends to continue to exist and will do what is in our power to guard and protect them;

We commit to spending time with our friends;

We share with our friends common choices and decisions centered in the effort to live virtuous lives; and

We share in our friends' joys and sorrows. (9.4.1)

Such a virtuous friendship includes both affirmation and admonition. We love the best that is within our friend and will therefore risk confronting our friend when he or she veers from the path of virtue. By contrast, within a friendship defined solely by utility or pleasure, we are reluctant to admonish, because "that's none of my business." Likewise, there will often be limits on how far we are willing to extend ourselves to an "incomplete" friend in need. If the friendship is primarily one of utility, we calculate the cost of our assistance; if it is rooted only in pleasure, we may distance ourselves when the relationship is no longer experienced as pleasurable. In a virtuous friendship we give of ourselves to the friend in need without counting the cost. Virtuous friends celebrate life's goodness together, stand by one another in times of challenge or loss, and seek the best for and from one another. Here is how Father Henri Nouwen (1997) expressed this: "Friendship is one of the greatest gifts a human being can receive. It is a bond beyond common goals, common interests, or common histories. It is a bond stronger than sexual union can create, deeper that a shared fate can solidify, and it can be more intimate than the bonds or marriage or community. Friendship is being with the other in joy and sorrow, even when we cannot increase the joy or decrease the sorrow. It is a unity of souls that gives nobility and sincerity to love. Friendship makes all of life shine brightly. Blessed are those who lay down their lives for their friends."[9]

What the Social Scientists Say about Friendship

Compared to Aristotle's vibrant descriptions of the virtues and responsibilities of friendship, the social scientific approach can sound dry and lifeless. It is ironic that those in the academy who are supposed to be most intimately acquainted with human psychology and social behavior sometimes shrink from the messiness of actual human lives and relationships. For example, Jon Nussbaum, a communications theorist who studies older adults' friendship, has written that "friendship is one relationship that most social scientists would rather not have to define" (1994, 210). Perhaps this is because friendship is, as sociologist Lillian Rubin described it, "a slippery subject at best—without institutional form, without a clearly defined set of norms for behavior or an agreed-upon set of reciprocal rights and obligations, without even any widely shared agreement about what is a friend" (Rubin 1981, quoted in Matthews 1986, 155).

On the other hand, even though social scientists often describe their quandary over definitions in the introductory sections of their papers about friendship and aging, they usually report that the aging persons they studied have no trouble whatsoever describing what they think a friend is. For example, Nussbaum described research he conducted in a retirement facility in Oklahoma. He and his colleagues interviewed residents, asking them questions like "What does friendship mean to you?" and "Has your view of friendship changed over the years?" (1994, 219). These elders described a complex vision of friendship, saying that it involved persons' devotion to one another over the course of many years and varying circumstances. They noted the importance of common interests, reciprocity, good communication, mutual respect and understanding. They also described a continuum of emotional closeness, and some felt that closeness was greater with friends than with family members. Finally, Nussbaum learned that these elders thought their lives would have been emotionally impoverished without friends. Nussbaum did not ask them whether they had read Aristotle, but their views are not all that far from his.

In another study of older men's and women's views on friendship, Rebecca Adams, Rosemary Blieszner, and Brian de Vries (2000) contacted people living in the southeastern United States and in western Canada and asked them to differentiate close and casual friends (U.S. sample) and to say what makes a person a friend or not a friend (Canadians). Most of the responses fell into a category the researchers labeled "behavioral processes." Adults ranging in age from 55 to 75 or older talked about how they shared personal information, did enjoyable things together, and helped one another in various ways. The "cognitive processes" identified by the researchers included loyalty, trust, shared values, empathy, and respect. Feelings of being comfortable together and caring for one another fell into the category of "affective processes." People indicated a sense of solidarity among their friends and also recognition of shared characteristics and roles such as widowhood; the authors labeled these the "structural" aspects of friendship. Finally, some differentiated close from casual friends by noting how long they had known the friend, the amount of contact they had, and whether the average duration of interactions went beyond, "Hi, how are you?" Many of the participants in this research talked about friendship using terms that fell into more than one of these categories. Again, they can be seen as describing Aristotelian categories of utility, pleasure, and virtue.

Given the large body of literature contrasting women's experiences of friendship with men's, it is not surprising that Adams, Blieszner, and de Vries (2000) found that the women in their study emphasized the emotional components of the relationship more than men, who were more likely to point to the "proxy" indicators, like length of time they had known someone and how much time they spent together.[10] One interesting finding emerging from this study was that the Canadians used more descriptors categorized as "affective" and "cognitive" than those in the United States, who tended to talk about friendship in terms of behaviors, along with the structural and proxy indicators. The take-home message from this research, as well as Nussbaum's, is that aging people have complex views of friendship, and they vary in the criteria they emphasize when thinking about what a friend is. In other words, they are not that much different from the gerontologists studying them.

Abiding Friendships

An old saying has it that you can choose your friends but you cannot choose your family. Aristotle would likely concur. It was his belief that one can sustain only a limited number of complete friendships, and it is therefore important to ascertain that another person shares your ideal of "the good" before committing to friendship. But if we take a few moments to reflect on our deepest and most abiding friendships we will likely discover that in many cases we cannot recall ever making a conscious choice to befriend the other. Often friendship, like life itself, just happens. Many people move in and out of our lives, but some friendships become richer, deeper, and more important over time. One way of thinking about this is to say that we do not choose such friendships so much as we receive them as a gift. As these friendships endure through time, we develop a common history, the story of our friendship. We laugh and cry together, share in one another's joys and sorrows, and watch one another's children grow into adulthood. Through these abiding friendships, we are granted good and faithful companions for life's journey, including the journey of aging.

Aging inevitably brings losses—weakened eyesight, diminished hearing, reduced mobility—along with accumulating aches and pains. Loved ones we have cherished pass to death. For many people, aging becomes a lonely journey as friendships based solely on utility or pleasure fade away. Those privileged to maintain loyal friendships as they journey together into old age are fortunate indeed. Memory becomes an important binder of friendship lived over time.

In long-time, intimate friendships, people celebrate life's milestones together—graduations, new jobs, weddings, births—and create a history of supporting one another in times of crisis and loss. Another way of saying this is that we have lived the story of our lives together. Sometimes we enjoy retelling stories out of our shared history—"remember the time we . . ."—but, spoken or not, these stories remind us of the bonds we share. As the passing years render the details of our stories hazy, we help each other to recall them: "No, that happened when we were in Boston." We know our own story better because we have entrusted a portion of our memory to our friends. We also come to realize that it really does not matter whether some shared experience happened in Boston. What is most important is the emotional residue of the connection experienced between friends. The *feelings* of friendship—love, loyalty, respect—are what the stories are really all about, and not the actual details of what happened when.

Because we have shared in a story lived over time, a friend can support us in a way that no one else can. If we turn to a "helping professional" in time of need, we often feel reduced to a "case" or "the 2:30 appointment"; a collection of symptoms rather than a person with a rich and complex life history. Our friends know our story, even the parts of our story that are hidden from us. We employ professional practitioners to address specific needs that demand their skill and expertise, but a friend can simply be present to us in our pain, fear, or grief. It is this gift of presence—sometimes without words and without recall of past experiences—that endures and nourishes friendships, especially when progressive forgetfulness enters the scene.

This question of what happens when dementia works its way into the bonds of friendship reverberates throughout all the chapters of this book and is addressed directly in the next chapter. The friend not struggling with memory loss can accept the responsibility for being the vessel holding memories. This can be critically important to family members and to paid workers if the friend is living in long-term care; a friend can remind these individuals about their lives, accomplishments, and gifts expressed before forgetfulness set in. Depending on the progression of the memory loss, having a friend who remembers shared experiences from the past can be a source of comfort and even entertainment. However, it may not always be helpful for the friend with intact memory to say to the one who is living with dementia, "Remember when . . ." The person may not remember, and being confronted with that loss can evoke anxiety. In that case, the friend must learn to enter the "now" of the relationship, to let go of concerns about recalling details about the past, and in loving relatedness, to enjoy taking a walk, breathing fresh air, listening to bird calls, painting a picture, singing a song, or just sitting quietly and occasionally squeezing each other's hands. Passing through the moment, the friend without dementia can recall the sharing of "now." There may be genuine grief for what has been lost, but it is to be hoped that the grief will be softened by gratitude for years of friendship and the feelings that remain.

CHAPTER FIVE

When Our Friends Travel the Dementia Road

Aristotle taught that virtuous friendship, like marriage, binds us to each other for better or worse, in sickness and in health. Inevitably, as we share the blessing of friendship through the process of aging, some friends we cherish (or we ourselves) will begin the journey of dementia. Dementia can challenge the ways in which we have previously experienced and understood our friendship. How do we continue to carry a portion of our friend's memory when she has lost much of her own portion of it? How can we be present to our friend when he no longer recognizes us or remembers our name? What happens when the "traveling hands of time" seem to be ticking away at two different speeds?

When someone sets out on the dementia road, incomplete friendships will likely come to an end in short order. As Aristotle noted, friendships based solely on utility assume that we will engage in mutually beneficial transactions. Thus, the person who is living with dementia may be perceived as no longer having value to offer in the relationship. Likewise, friendships grounded only in pleasure will likely not endure when the friend who has dementia no longer engages with the themes and interests we shared. It does not always bring pleasure to spend time with someone who has dementia, particularly as the condition progresses. One by one friendships based on utility or pleasure fade away, with people often mumbling words to the effect of "Pete has already left us; I would rather remember him as he was."

Life spans are increasing. Medical science has become more effective in curing or treating various life-threatening diseases. Inevitably, more people within our social convoy—including cherished friends and family members in the innermost circle—will receive the dreaded diagnosis. We will need to learn not only how to offer them our strength and support but also how to continue to share a rich, mutually enjoyable friendship during this new stage of the aging journey. Some would object that true friendship cannot be maintained within dementia because friendship must always include *reciprocity*, and they cannot imagine what the person who has dementia has to offer as a friend. One of us once described to an acquaintance the joy found in sharing the company of persons who are living with advanced dementia. She replied with a quizzical look, "I understand how they benefit, but what do you get out of it?"

Such a perspective on friendship reflects the values of a materialistic culture, which counts another person's worth only in terms of what he or she can offer that has value to us or the wider society. This perspective assumes that if we give of ourselves in friendship, we should expect something in return. But while reciprocity is indeed a component of friendship, it is not a continuous reality. We may pass through a difficult period in life when our emotional or physical resources are limited, and we can but gratefully accept the gift of our friend's support and encouragement. At another time, these roles may reverse. Friendship lived over time places reciprocity into a broader framework than that of a simple, time-bound transaction. It means being present to a friend in a given moment without weighing the costs and benefits.

We should not underestimate the gifts that a friend who has dementia may offer. That friend may well serve as a teacher, offering lessons in what it is to be a person, what gives life value and worth, and how the meaning and importance of friendship are not bounded by cognition. A friend who has dementia may also teach valuable lessons in what constitutes genuine joy and fulfillment. Dementia does not reduce friendship to a one-way street. Rather, it can introduce us to new dimensions of what makes for a good and worthwhile life in ways that help us to overcome the limits imposed by our own fears. If it is indeed our relationships with others that make us a self, a friend who has dementia may help us grow into deeper understandings of our own selfhood.

It is worthwhile to return to Aristotle's five features of a "complete" friendship to consider which elements change and which remain the same when one of us develops dementia. *We wish good for our friends and seek to do good on their behalf.* We wish for our friend who has dementia to enjoy the fullest possible experience of life. Therefore, we will do what we can to help our friend attain and remain within his or her "joy zone."

We first heard the idea of a joy zone described by a much-beloved geriatrician who came rushing into a conference on palliative care to give a presentation on end-of-life care for persons who have advanced dementia. Barely stopping to catch her breath, she launched into this story of how her day had begun long before sunrise:

> I came down the stairs and received an immediate emotional lift. The night before I had cut peonies in my garden and put them into a vase, and I could smell them from the landing. It is my favorite smell in the world, and I immedi-

ately put that into my "dementia toolbox." All of us should be stocking that toolbox with the things that put us into our "joy zone" and telling our spouse or loved ones about them. If we live long enough, either my husband or I will someday become the other's caregiver. If I am the one who has dementia, I want him to know what will bring me joy. If I am living with dementia, I want to smell fresh peonies whenever possible. And I want to hear a baseball game on the radio. This is funny, because I do not like baseball. But the sound of a game on the radio always takes me back to my girlhood and summer nights on the front porch with my father. So I want to hear a baseball game on the radio. It could be the same game, over and over; I probably won't notice that. I just want to hear the sound of the game and smell the peonies.

If short-term memory has become problematic, we may make use of our experience of common story to find the points of reference with which our friend can still engage. We offer specific suggestions on doing this in Chapter 11. For now, we simply want to note that stories of happy events from the past, whether remembered clearly or dimly, can still bring animation and engagement. Because we know our friend's story intimately, we know his or her passions and interests—gardening, cooking, woodworking, knitting—and can lift up these passions through either recollection or active pursuit in the present. We know our friend's tastes in music and art and bring these "joy zone" elements into our friend's environment. As a friend, we have unique resources to offer that no professional caregiver can duplicate. Out of the depth of our knowledge of our friend, we can provide things that bring peace and pleasure through the cloud of anxiety and confusion that so often accompanies dementia. And because we experience our own selfhood in relationship with our friend, his or her joy becomes our joy as well. Indeed, our friend may give us new gifts of joy, exposing the lie that such friendship is a one-way street.

We want our friends to continue to exist and will do what is in our power to guard and protect them. "Continued existence" as a goal moves us into the complex world of medical ethics and the circumstances under which continued mortal existence has value and meaning. But "guarding and protecting" speaks of the role of advocate, a critical role for a friend when a cherished person is living within the reality of dementia. Even when there is a dedicated care partner, the maze that must be navigated to gain access to needed services can be overwhelming. As our friend's advocate, we can join family members in insisting that these services be made available. Because families may not have time, energy, or expertise to engage in advocacy (which may involve repeated contacts with various institutions and organizations), we can care for our friend by taking on this important responsibility.

The goodness of life and the fullest experience of personhood are found in our relationships with others in community, especially relationships with friends. Dementia does not reduce a friend to an "it," and the challenges it brings call for more engagement from friends, not less. When we view dementia as a private matter—a problem to be addressed only by family members, medical practitioners, and professional caregivers—we undercut the core of our friend's selfhood and our own.

We commit to spending time with our friends. The greatest gift of friendship is our presence, and this is particularly true when our friend travels the dementia road. Too often visits from friends become both briefer and less frequent as dementia progresses—courtesy calls rather than meaningful time together. Regular visits increase the likelihood that we will be recognized, perhaps not by name, but recognized nonetheless, as one who brings gifts of peace, comfort, and joy. Through frequent visits, we will learn what causes our friend distress or agitation and what creates and sustains the joy zone. We will learn new ways to enjoy the goodness of our friendship.

It is common and understandable that people try to deny permission for the person they cherish to travel the dementia road. They want their friend back as he or she was, attempting to recreate his or her former cognitive state through continuous efforts to orient and stimulate memory. "Hi, Fred! Do you know who I am? What day is it? What did you have for breakfast?" Such efforts rarely succeed and often create anxiety. Friends are called to be present to persons who have dementia, focusing on what can be enjoyed together in the present rather than attempting to recover what was shared in the past. "Hi, Fred! It's Bill, your friend. I've come to spend some time with you. You're looking well today!"

Presence can take many forms, including sitting in silence together, taking a walk, listening to music, playing a game, looking at photographs, or reminiscing about shared history. These are precisely the things that any two friends might do together. As people spend time in the company of friends who have dementia, they can discover that friendship remains very much a two-way street, with each giving and receiving gifts, just as in the past. Some of the gifts received from a friend who has memory loss will be continuous with those received in the past, while others will be new and different.

Common images of dementia in general and Alzheimer's disease in particular tend to be profoundly negative and reductionist. People who have Alzheimer's become mean. People who have Alzheimer's alternate between shouting and mumbling incoherently. People who have Alzheimer's stare into space and do not communicate. And to be sure, all of these descriptions characterize at least some persons some of the time. We have no desire to romanticize a condition that can bring great pain to those living with it as well as those who love them. There may well be days when friends cannot successfully engage and their presence brings agitation rather than peace. But in what friendship is this not true? The next visit may bring a very different experience.

Within dementia there is both continuity of the personality and significant change as a person lives less within the cognitive self and more within the emotional self. People are often greatly distressed to witness this change, because modern Western society equates "self" so strongly with cognition: adults are to conduct themselves rationally, maintain control over emotions, and choose their words with care. Dementia can bring the loss of impulse control and allow the direct expression of emotions—anger, joy, love—that people have been long conditioned to "keep a lid on." As we noted in Chapter 3, Alzheimer's disease and other forms of dementia significantly challenge our taken-for-granted assumptions of what it means to be an adult, what it is to be a "self."

It is also true that dementia can bring a new and delightful spontaneity. As a geriatric psychiatrist once expressed it, "My friends who have Alzheimer's come up with the best one-liners!" Friends who previously tended to be reserved and formal may become eager for physical touch—hugs and kisses—and more open in expressing gratitude and affection. After a visit with her mother, who had advanced dementia, a woman said in wonder, "I have received more kisses from Mom this week alone that I received in my entire childhood." Friends may become less inhibited. The woman who previously permitted no "cuss words" under her roof may take to swearing like a sailor. Her friends may choose to be appalled, or they may choose to be amused and delighted by the salty talk she now gives herself permission to use. In spending time with friends, people come to understand and appreciate that living primarily within the emotional self can be as rich and full an expression of personhood as living primarily within the cognitive self. We value and enjoy our friend as he or she is in the present. We spend time with our friend, not as an act of charity, but as the continuation of a friendship we both still value and enjoy.

We share with our friends common choices and decisions centered in the effort to live virtuous lives. Aristotle likely could not have imagined this dimension of friendship continuing when one friend develops dementia, because his understanding of virtue was defined by conscious, rational choices to pursue "the good." But as long as people continue to share in relationships with others and participate in the fabric of community, they have opportunities to make virtuous choices. The fundamental expressions of virtue—kindness, consideration, sharing, gratitude, forgiveness—are less an expression of cognitive choice than of an essential emotional posture toward life and other people. Those who have been privileged to spend time in a memory care section within a nursing home experience a complex set of social relationships, which Lauren Kessler (2007) describes as "a vibrant community of quirky souls" (11), with the full range of personalities that one would find in any community of similar size. So long as we live in community with others, we have the opportunity to continue our growth in virtuous living.

Our friend who is traveling the dementia road will inevitably challenge us to reconsider prior assumptions about what constitutes a life of virtue. Our friend may, for example, help us learn such virtues as humility, patience, and living fully in the present moment. He or she may also inspire us to think in new ways about what gives our own life meaning, worth, and value, particularly if we have looked almost exclusively to productivity and autonomy for their source. The heart of virtue lies in recognizing and honoring the inherent dignity and worth of each fellow human being without regard for that person's abilities or achievements. Sharing in friendship with a person on the journey of dementia teaches important lessons about the heart of virtue.

We share in our friends' joy and sorrow. If our friend is now living primarily out of the emotional self, both sorrow and joy may be experienced more deeply and expressed more fully than before. Many of us have spent our lives attempting to use reason to temper the extremes of life's highs and life's lows by placing them into "proper perspective." There is value in the effort to keep life on an even keel, but there is also a cost to be paid when we do not permit ourselves to fully experience either distress or enjoyment. To be fully present to a friend who has dementia means that we will weep, sometimes uncontrollably, but also that we may laugh more uproariously than we have permitted ourselves to do in many years. Virtuous friendship means carrying each other's sorrow and sharing each other's joy, as Nouwen expressed it, "even when we cannot increase the joy or decrease the sorrow." This is the heart of being present as a friend, accompanying our cherished friend in his or her journey of dementia.

Tests of Friendship

Even a virtuous friendship such as Aristotle described will be tested. Reflecting on how dementia can invade the space between friends offers many examples of such tests, especially when the responses of a person who has memory loss do not fit our ideals of friendly interaction. Add in various problems like hearing loss and the physical relocation of the person who has dementia to a dementia-care facility, and it is easy to see how such a relationship can undergo what Sarah Matthews (1986) called a "turning." Obviously, death is the major "turning" for the termination of friendship. Few of the healthy older people Matthews interviewed terminated friendships intentionally. Instead, some friendships simply faded away when one friend had fewer financial resources for shared activities, a lack of transportation prevented face-to-face contact, or the onset of dementia disrupted expectations about communication and the rhythm of two people interacting. In one of the earliest sociological writings on friendship in later life, Beth Hess (1972) observed that what makes friendships so meaningful—they are voluntary—also makes them vulnerable to breakage. We do not choose our families, but we can choose to enter into friendship with others, although in many cases it may seem less like a deliberate choice than a kind of drifting into relationship.

In an early paper on the strains in older people's friendships, Karen Rook (1989) noted that because so many social roles change or disappear as we grow older, we need our friends even more as a grounding for our sense of self. However, friendships have social costs that can sometimes be troubling. For example, a relationship can be ruptured when a friend fails to repay a loan (an act of omission) or says something nasty about you behind your back (an act of commission). As Rook wrote, friends can "violate norms of trust, respect, reciprocity, and status equality" (1989, 171). There can also be violations of norms that are peculiar to the friendship. These include unspoken agreements about topics that will not be discussed. Then there are the problems caused when an effort to help a friend backfires. We may think we are offering helpful instrumental or emotional support, but the casserole delivered in a pot that needs to be returned or the chatty telephone call that comes just as the nice warm bath is beckoning with a few minutes of quiet solitude may not be appreciated. The person who lives with progressive forgetfulness can be on either side of these transactions.

Rook (1989) offered a long list of possible problems in lengthy friendships. Sometimes there is a lack of agreement about a comfortable level of intimacy and self-disclosure. One person in the relationship might value spontaneity—stopping by for a cup of coffee—while the other person keeps a calendar and likes to have predictable, planned social encounters. Then there is the "seeing the mote in the other person's eye" problem, when the log in your own goes unnoticed. This can definitely strain a relationship to the breaking point as, for example, when a person with a long history of strained and difficult parent-child relationships gives advice on managing interactions with an adult child. Psychologists call this *projection* (the unconscious process of casting my problems onto you), but by whatever name it is called, it can be toxic for friendship.

Rook's list continued with the problematic personality characteristics that cause a "turning" in a friendship in later life. The person who relishes "dishing dirt" may finally drive another person away when the poison of cruel gossip takes the relationship to its tipping point. Problems with a friend's social network (especially family members) can also cause cleavages. Recall, for example, the distress of the woman we described in the Introduction who called us because of what a person in her bowling group had said about her husband, who has a form of dementia.

Finally, Rook noted that external events, like a change in financial status, widowhood, or divorce, or a disruptive health problem can all create problems in friendships. Adding to this challenging vision of late-life friendship is the observation that these problems can interact, making us feel, by the time we finish reading Rook's paper, somewhat amazed that any friendships can survive the journey into old age. Surely the fact that they do, and that many become more precious with each passing year, is a testimony to the resilience of the human spirit.

What do older people do in response to these strains on friendship? Interviews of elderly women by Moremen (2008) revealed strains similar to those identified earlier by Rook. Moremen argued that the primary reason for problems in friendships was the disruption of expectations. The women she spoke with expected their friends to be trustworthy and honest, and sometimes this expectation was violated. These women assumed that their friends would share similar interests, but the activities that interest people can lose their allure. Moremen's interviewees did not want their friends to be overly dependent or "whiney" about their problems, but sometimes they were. In these and other ways, Moremen found older women feeling that their friends did not live up to their expectations. And what did they do about these strains? Not much. They wanted to avoid conflict, so they simply drifted away from contact with people whom they had formerly counted as friends.

The observations of Rook, Moremen, and other social scientists who have studied strains in long-term friendships lead us to return to Aristotle's five features of a virtuous friendship.[1] Earlier we reflected on them from the perspective of the individual whose friend has begun the journey into dementia, and we noted many ways that a friendship might be tested when someone's responses to other people and the environment become disordered. However, it is also important to consider these features from the other side of the relationship and to ask how the individual who has memory loss might experience these signs of friendship in a positive or negative manner.

The first two features—seeking to do good for the other and attempting to guard and protect her or him—may be perceived as intrusive and paternalistic, especially by the individual who has just begun to adjust to life with memory loss. In a later work detailing her research on older adults' friendship, Sarah Matthews (1996) concluded that "the only circumstance that apparently leads to loss of friends is becoming frail, dependent, and/or housebound" (412). She related this to American social norms about reciprocity in friendship and stated that "when one friend becomes dependent on the goodwill of the other, he or she may act to limit interaction to avoid harming the relationship" (416).

Karen Roberto described this as feeling "overbenefitted" (1996, 67), and she found that those who experienced this feeling were less content and happy with their friendships. In other words, persons who are becoming increasingly challenged by memory loss and perhaps other assorted physical problems may not want to accept a friend's efforts to do good for them and protect them from harm. They might, instead, feel overbenefitted—forced into a relationship that feels inappropriately one-sided. Not everyone has the ability to tolerate receiving more than can be given. In this case, it is usually incumbent on the individual who is not experiencing progressive forgetfulness to be sensitive to the friend's potential for feeling overbenefitted and to find ways to offer reassurance that the relationship still has the potential for mutuality.

People who are living with memory loss are often described as having a sixth sense about emotion. Talk to any CNA (certified nursing assistant) working with persons who have dementia and you will hear tales of how the residents can pick up on subtle cues about their emotional state. For example, a CNA may come to work feeling fretful about a child's school problems or a romantic entanglement. Trying to put on a happy face, she will soon discover that the morning "cares" for Mrs. Jones (e.g., toileting, face washing, tooth brushing) do not go well because Mrs. Jones has noted the cues of her distress.

In 1978, Frances Hellenbradt, a retired professor of physical medicine living in a retirement community in Ohio, published an insightful brief reflection on "the senile dement in our midst." She described how the facility where she lived had established what today we would call a dementia-care unit, but in 1978, it was called the Convalarium. It embraced the "new culture" of care long before Tom Kitwood defined it by focusing on "residual abilities, not losses" (1997, 68).

Reflecting on the emotional receptivity of people who are living with dementia, even in the later stages, Hillebrandt commented that the Convalarium "is no place for 'do-gooders'; an insincere approach is so infallibly discerned by the patient as to suggest that some important aspects of personality and spirit do not reside in those parts of the brain that atrophy in senile dementia" (1978, 68).

In her portrayal of working as a CNA at a residence for persons who had dementia, English professor Lauren Kessler (2007) provided several examples of this ability to read the emotions of another person from facial expression, voice, and physical interaction. One of Kessler's stories speaks not just of sensitivity to the emotions of others but of friendship between two people who had advanced dementia. Eloise was having a bad day, insisting she wanted to go HOME. Kessler, her CNA for the day, tried everything she could think of to distract her, but this only seemed to increase her distress. Finally, after Eloise had been yelling for some time about wanting to go home, another resident—Dottie, whose room was next door—assessed the situation and took over. Dottie told Eloise to come in her room to make a phone call to her daughter in Chicago. They sat on Dottie's bed, holding the phone, while Dottie randomly punched in numbers. Was Dottie deliberately engaging in the pretense of making the call? Kessler did not know, but what she did see was that Eloise began to calm down. "It doesn't seem to matter that the call is not going through, that Dottie is just pressing random buttons. Eloise is involved in this moment with her friend. She is sitting on her bed having a little talk with Dottie. Her anxiety ebbs" (126). Later, they emerged from Dottie's room and Kessler made them both a cup of tea.

As a caveat to this discussion, we need to recall the description of the different types of dementia. Research in the 1990s that did not differentiate types of dementia (or referred broadly to "dementia of the Alzheimer type") found little difference between persons who are living with the diagnosis and "normal controls" in recognition of facial expressions of emotion.[2] A more recent study of persons identified as having Alzheimer's dementia suggested that differences between their ability to recognize emotions and those of the persons in the control group reflected problems not in emotion recognition but rather in the ways their brains' visual and spatial processing systems functioned when they observed pictures showing various facial expressions (Burnham and Hogervorst 2004). Further, because of so many more different forms of dementia being diagnosed today, clinicians are beginning to observe that some may bring greater impairment in recognizing emotions in others. This appears to be especially true of persons who have frontotemporal dementia (Rosen et al. 2004). In reviewing research like this and trying to connect it to the anecdotal reports of

CNAs, it is important to recognize that this research usually asks people to look at pictures of faces of strangers displaying various emotional expressions (like anger, fear, happiness, sadness). The CNA who notes that Mrs. Jones seems to know that she is having a bad day is present in multiple ways to Mrs. Jones in a relationship. There are visual cues of the whole body and not just the face, along with vocal cues and tactile cues. Thus, Mrs. Jones might in some way ascertain that she is being washed rather harshly on the day that Mary, the CNA, just broke up with her boyfriend.

We took this digression into talking about how persons perceive others' emotions because of two of Aristotle's other points about virtuous friendships. He said that in these relationships, people commit to spending time with their friends, but what matters is not the time itself, but what transpires during the time spent with a friend who has dementia. If we stop by for a visit to a person living in his home or in some kind of dementia-care setting and appear to be nervous or impatient or in some way uncomfortable, it is likely that our friend will note this, if not consciously, then at some deeper, nonconscious, even bodily level. Moreover, our efforts to share common choices and decisions may be perceived not as common but as imposed, serving as one more reminder of the confusing world wrought by forgetfulness.

Emotions can be contagious, and because the ability to reason has been compromised, the individual who has dementia may have few defenses against "catching" another person's negative emotions. Persons without dementia also experience emotion contagion, but they can (sometimes) rely on rational attributions, such as "my friend seems agitated because he just found out the IRS is auditing him" or "my friend's always a little anxious; that's just how he is." Many books written for those caring for persons who are living with dementia address this issue, including the classic and revered *The 36-Hour Day*, which is now in its fourth edition, having first appeared in 1981, when there were few resources for family members struggling with all the complex challenges of caring for a loved one who has dementia. Regarding the problem of emotion contagion, the authors wrote: "Even people with a severe dementia remain sensitive to the moods of people around them. If there is tension in the household, no matter how well you try to conceal it, the person may respond to it" (Mace and Rabins 2006, 154).

Aristotle's last observation about virtuous friendship—sharing joys and sorrows—can also test relationships and values about social interactions. Recognizing that all persons who are living with dementia are living with it in their own ways, grounded in their own life histories and expressing their own unique personalities, we need to tread carefully here. How much emotion censoring should we engage in when we are with our friend? If I am feeling sorrow, should I stay away so I do not take a chance on spreading it, or does that decision devalue the relationship and the person? If I am feeling joy, should I stay away so that my friend who has few opportunities to encounter that which has caused my joy will not feel deprived?

We have no easy answers to these questions and note that they arise not only in our friendships with persons who have dementia but in all friendships. Friendship always involves risks. Much that transpires between two persons in close relationships cannot be controlled. But, if we enter into the relationship aware of our own foibles and needs and with an open heart toward the other, we usually will be all right. With that perspective, we often find that our friend who has dementia, whose self-censoring mechanism has broken down because of the loss of higher-order cognition, gifts us with this feature of virtuous friendship by purely presenting us with both joy and sorrow.

Friendship can be hard. It is tested, not only on the grade school playground and the halls of the middle school, but all through life. As people get older, they may find some relationships more sorely tested and choose to distance themselves from certain persons "in the convoy." The literature on older adult friendships amply documents these tests. In addition, a large body of empirical research shows that with age comes the increasing motivation to regulate emotion in favor of positive experiences. One study even showed that compared to younger adults, older people looking at pictures of faces fixated more on smiles than on frowns (Isaacowitz et al. 2006). This is not to say that older adults *cannot* experience sadness, fear, anger, and other emotions that sometimes get labeled as "negative." However, with age comes the increasing desire to structure life whenever possible to experience rewarding emotions rather than troubling ones.

For more than two decades, Stanford University psychologist Laura Carstensen and her colleagues have conducted research on aging people's choices to spend time with those who "maximize social and emotional gains and minimize social and emotional risks" (1992, 331). Usually these are close friends and family members. As people get older and realize on some level that their time is limited, they choose not to invest energy in new relationships, troubling ones, or those based only on gaining information. This behavior is predicted by Carstensen's "socioemotional selectivity theory," a rich source of testable hypotheses about the nature of close relationships across the life span and how the awareness of limited time affects them. More recently, Carstensen and colleagues have been studying the experience of poignancy, that blend of positive and negative emotions that washes over us like a wave when we know that a good experience (or relationship) will inevitably come to an end (Ersner-Hershfield et al. 2008).

Currently, there is little empirical research documenting how persons who are living with dementia regulate emotionality through their choices about social interactions; nor do we have studies of how they experience poignancy. One study of nursing home residents who were described as being cognitively intact enough to "to give reasonable and consistent responses to interview questions" (Powers 1996, 181) found that residents developed various ways to ward off interactions with other residents who upset them by invading their privacy and being overly demanding. In contrast, they also were able to identify persons whose companionship they welcomed. In other words, they were expressing "socioemotional selectivity."

In the emerging autobiographical literature on "early-stage dementia" describing persons still living independently, we find many expressions of people's grief over the impact of the diagnosis on close relationships and the intimations of losses to come. For example, Richard Taylor's (2007) intimate descriptions of his experiences of living with Alzheimer's disease testify to this. He writes: "The locus of my attention is definitely shifting from my head to my heart. I feel and think about feelings more than I think about thinking. I feel sad, and mad, and happy, and grateful, I feel loved, ignored, needed, and like a dying albatross that is chained around each of the people who cares about me. Sometimes I'm very happy, and sometimes I'm very sad, and at all times I am aware of all my feelings" (128).

Taylor and the other courageous persons who have written about their experiences of dementia reveal much about the tests of friendship from the perspective of persons living with forgetfulness.[3] Within these accounts, one can find indications that they are demonstrating "socioemotional selectivity" because they restrict interactions with persons they experience as distressing.

Responding to the Tests of Friendship

In the last section, we claimed that late-life friendships can be tested for those with and without the dementia diagnosis. Although we are not aware of any research to confirm this, we suspect that some people are probably better able to cope with these tests. For example, we know a man we will call Steve, who has faithfully remained a friend to Charlie for more than forty years. Over the last decade, Charlie has gradually lost more and more aspects of cognitive functioning, and he now lives in a residence for persons who have dementia. Charlie's wife died a few years ago and they had no children. Before the dementia progressed and he could no longer live independently, Charlie asked Steve to be his legal guardian, a responsibility Steve accepted. Steve has faithfully visited Charlie in his new living environment, but a few weeks ago, on an autumn Saturday afternoon when he expected to watch a college football game with his friend, Steve encountered Charlie in an agitated state. Charlie shouted at him and told him not to come back, saying he was bothering him and that he did not want to see him anymore.

Steve was devastated by this experience. He could have responded in several ways. For example, he might have said to himself, "well, if that's the way you show gratitude for all I've done for you, you can find yourself a new guardian because I'm out of here." Or, he might have fretted about what terrible thing he might have unknowingly done to his friend to elicit such a reaction. Fearing future encounters like that and needing to regulate his own emotional state, he might have chosen to disengage from Charlie. But Steve did none of these things. Instead, he attributed Charlie's response to the fact that, like all people, he was "having a bad day" and trusted that in the next encounter, the relationship would be repaired. Because of his legal standing with Charlie, he did not have to be concerned about HIPAA (Health Insurance Portability and Accountability Act) regulations about privacy and thus could inquire of the CNA in Charlie's residence about whether anything had happened that might have upset him that day. It turned out that he had awakened not feeling well and about thirty minutes before Steve showed up, two other residents had been shouting at each other.

Why would one person respond to a test of friendship with anger, another with anxiety, and still another with understanding and compassion? Clues to this can be found in thinking about the different ways people form friendships and the security or insecurity people feel about relationships.

There have been many efforts in the friendship literature to categorize friendships, but one that is particularly relevant to our topic is the approach of Sarah Matthews, who conducted over sixty lengthy interviews with older people between the ages of 60 and 80 about their experiences of friendship. From these interviews, Matthews identified three friendship styles. The *independent* style of friendship describes people whose high expectations for friends never seemed to be met. These individuals knew a lot of people and did not consider them-selves to be isolated in any way; they just could not cite specific persons they thought of as friends. Matthews said they seemed to be "surrounded by a sea of people, none distinguished from others" (1986, 45). In a later work, Matthews observed that persons with this independent style would be "out of luck" (1996, 425) when frailty set in, for just as they had developed no enduring commit-ments to others, others had not developed commitments to them. Persons in the second category—the *discerning*—could name a few close friendships cultivated and nurtured over many years. On the other hand, these individuals also noted persons who had not accompanied their social convoy into old age. Matthews called her third friendship style *acquisitive,* depicting persons who easily made new friends while also maintaining old friendships. They were open to others and seemed to have spent their lives "collecting a variety of friendships" (53).

Steve would probably classify himself as discerning. Like the people Mat-thews described in that group, he had a long history of relationships with a few good friends, friends he expected to keep until death. He did not expect to add new friends to his "convoy" but was content to be loyal and steadfast with the persons he had connected with many years ago.

In terms of attachment theory, which we discussed in Chapter 3, Steve would probably also be described by some psychologists as having a secure attachment style. He does not worry about whether Charlie is still his friend. Although hurt and upset by Charlie's outburst, he could easily attribute it to what psychologists call "situational variables" and not to malice or deliberate rejection by Charlie. As we learned in Chapter 3, attachment theory offers a perspective on human relationships across the life span. People with preoccupied, dismissing, or fear-ful styles of attachment will have more difficulty navigating many aspects of friendship in old age, particularly those that are colored by dementia. We are not, however, making a deterministic argument here, and we do not mean to imply that it would be impossible for an insecurely attached person to remain in friendship with someone who is living with dementia.

Continuing in friendship with some persons can be challenging, both for the individual who has dementia and for the one experiencing no troublesome memory loss or confusion. This is true regardless of individual personality pro-files, the history of the relationship, and the current situation. Socioemotional selectivity theory says that people grow more selective about emotional invest-ments in relationships as they grow older. We may simply have less emotional energy to invest in friendship, especially as we experience our own burdens of aging: accumulating chronic illnesses, losses of loved ones, reduced engagement with the world. At this point, we may realize that we need the support of others in navigating the terrain of late-life friendship. Another way of saying this is that all of us—persons with and without the dementia diagnosis—need a flourishing community for support in sustaining and even growing our friendships with one another as we grow older.

CHAPTER SIX

Dementia Fear and Anxiety

An imagined monologue:

> OK, OK. So you already told me about different kinds of dementia and what it's
> like to hear the doctor say, "You probably have Alzheimer's." I know that other
> people are important to us and that I should be grateful for my family and my
> friends. I do my best to stay in touch with friends, but you know, it's hard
> these days with so many pressures on my time. My friend, Mary, doesn't
> seem to be doing so well right now. She's a few years older than I am and she
> doesn't seem as sharp as she used to be. She calls me sometimes and talks
> about the same things in every conversation. At the end of the call, she repeats
> what she said at the beginning, as if she has no clue we'd already discussed those
> things. And, yes, I know you think that people need to stick together in communi-
> ties and that we should get over our pride and learn to depend on one another.
> I hear that sometimes in church, though of course I'm so busy that it's hard to
> get there regularly. You know something? To be perfectly honest, all this stuff
> sounds good, but you don't understand. . . . I've had a few memory lapses lately.
> I have three children, and sometimes when I'm with them, I feel like they're
> checking me out. I'm terrified I'll forget something or repeat myself in front of
> them. In fact, my daughter has started bugging me to see my doctor. I'm scared
> of what he might tell me. What if I have it, like I think my friend, Mary, does?
> What will happen to me?

In 1948, the year we were born, W. H. Auden's long poem *The Age of Anxiety*
won the Pulitzer Prize for poetry. Although the postwar years "boomed" with a
high birth rate and economic growth (at least in the United States), Auden's
naming of the times rang true for many people. Existentialism's stark, unapolo-
getic vision of the human condition reverberated through philosophy, literature,
and the social sciences, and some said the fruits of its critique of social structures (especially political and religious ones) ripened in the streets of protest in
the late '60s.

Now, those who took to the streets, and their brothers and sisters who did not,
are living into an old age that is fraught with a new form of anxiety: whether
memory and cognitive fitness can be preserved until death. These are the people

who merrily sang along with the band members of the Who (whose surviving members are now in their sixties) as they boldly declared, "hope I die before I get old." Now, they are saying, "hope I die before I get dementia." We have heard variations on this phrase when we tell people who are our age about this book. Sometimes, it seems as if they take a figurative step backward from us, as if even thinking about this topic might be infectious. Even more troubling are descriptions given by persons who are living with the diagnosis. Several have told us about walking into a room where people know about their diagnosis and seeing them move away. We have also heard how individuals diagnosed with a form of dementia are told by well-meaning friends, "Oh, I forget things, too." In other words, to defend themselves against dementia fear and anxiety, people sometimes minimize its impact on those who are already traveling the dementia road.

The very word *dementia* has become controversial because of the emotional freight associated with it. We were surprised by the strong reaction of a friend who asked about this book and was told the title referred to dementia. "You can't do that," she objected. "No one will want to read your book!"

In a study conducted in Great Britain, people in the early stage of dementia described their negative reactions to the word *dementia* because it called up images of being "demented." They stated no more positive feelings about the term *Alzheimer's disease*, as they did not feel "diseased" (Langdon, Eagle, and Warner 2007). Researchers need to be cautious about the terms they use when they recruit people to participate in research. Because many are sensitive to the stigma associated with the diagnosis, some researchers are now using the phrase "memory impairment" (Clare, Goater, and Woods 2006).

To be fair, we should note that baby boomers are not the only ones who worry about dementia. Older adults grimly joke about "parts-heimer's" disease, and young adults taking courses on aging sometimes express their own anxieties about dementia, particularly if they have watched as a grandparent journeyed into the land of forgetfulness. All these persons may also experience the kind of anxiety Auden depicted when they reflect on the myriad worries of the postmodern psyche (the economy, the environment, the threat of terrorist attacks, etc.), but somehow the threat of dementia seems more personal. We have relationships with people who have Alzheimer's and other forms of memory loss, and we know that their stories are all associated with aging and will all end with death. Although much hope is currently being invested in biomedical science to "find a cure" for Alzheimer's disease and other dementias, there is no cure for mortality—nor for aging (despite the claims of "antiaging medicine").

In 2006, the MetLife Foundation released a study using a nationally representative sample of 1,008 adults that showed Americans 55 or older fearing Alzheimer's more than any other disease, including cancer.[1] Generalizing from this sample, the researchers concluded that more than one-third of adults in the United States have a family member or friend who has Alzheimer's, and about 60 percent worry that they may someday have to care for someone who has dementia. Sibyl Jacobson, president and CEO of the MetLife Foundation, expressed concern that less than 20 percent of Americans so worried about dementia had "done anything to prepare for a disease that destroys a person's memory, personality, and ability to function independently." Statements like this make it hardly surprising that many people simply do not want to think about dementia, nor about the possibility that they or persons they care about will one day receive the diagnosis.

In 2009, approximately the same number of Americans were surveyed about their knowledge of Alzheimer's disease and their experiences with persons having the diagnosis. More than a third of those people who participated in the telephone survey stated that they worry about "getting Alzheimer's."[2] Research conducted in England that involved interviews with people age 60 or older who were not caring for a person who had dementia and had not received the diagnosis themselves reached similar conclusions: (1) people do not have much information about progressive memory loss; (2) they are fearful about "tipping over" from normal forgetting into dementia (especially if they know someone who has the diagnosis); and (3) their anxiety centers on "a perceived loss of independence, control, identity, and dignity" (Corner and Bond 2004, 150).

In her brilliantly titled book *Forget Memory*, Anne Basting asks this question: "To what extent do our fears about dementia and aging contribute to the tragic conditions of living with dementia and the catastrophic economic story of dementia?" (2009, 2–3). In no way does she dismiss these fears as unfounded. She knows how real they are and the toll they take on individual lives, and she sympathizes with people who feel this fear so acutely. While viewing aspects of the fear as natural because of dementia's association with loss and death, she also notes the many ways in which the fear is amplified. Her book analyzes how novels, films, television shows, and other forms of the popular media weave a story of dementia that is mostly dark and tragic. This serves the purposes of organizations competing for private and public support in the fundraising arena of America life. Not only do the stories of tragic loss "tug at the heartstrings" of donors, but the commodification of dementia through the repeated refrain of how much it costs the U.S. economy today and how much it will cost in the future (a refrain echoed in other countries as well) also feeds the fear reverberating through the culture.

And what do people fear? Basting asked people, and they listed some of the fears we mentioned in earlier chapters. Above all, the greatest fear is being a burden to others. With autonomy and independence widely viewed as essential to adult well-being, no one wants to deny that well-being to persons they love by burdening them with caregiving responsibilities. Dementia also elicits fear of the unknown: "Am I next? Is my forgetting normal or pathological?" People fear losing control over their lives, for having a form of dementia means that some-day safe driving will not be possible, and others will have to make decisions about basic aspects of life. Basting also heard stories of the fear of having to hand over a lifetime of savings to paid caregivers rather than passing a financial legacy to others. Finally, because our culture has largely rejected cosmic or transcen-dent sources of meaning for old age and has eliminated much social and com-munal support for late-life meaning (Cole 1992; Moody 1986), people are left to their own devices to secure a sense of meaningfulness. This might work as long as physical and mental well-being remain, but when the illusion of autonomy can no longer be maintained because of progressive forgetfulness and confu-sion, then life may seem to lose its meaning and purpose.

While never dismissing the fear or demeaning the people who feel it, Basting weaves a new story about dementia, a story of joy, love, and hope located not in anticipation of a medical cure for dementia but in the kinds of relationships we can have with people who can no longer remember who we are. We need to "forget memory" because memory is not the whole story of a meaningful human life. In fact, in a series of colorful, eye-catching posters that celebrate the publica-tion of the book, she proclaimed, "Forget memory. Try imagination!" *Forget Memory* documents a variety of ways people—with and without the diagnosis of dementia—can connect interpersonally through creative activities that stimu-late the imagination and do not rely on memory or even language. We will have more to say about creativity in a later chapter, when we describe specific ways friends can enter and enjoy the "joy zone" together.

In the last few paragraphs, we alternated between talking about fear and about anxiety. There are important differences between fear and anxiety, and people experience *both* in response to dementia. As we work through our discus-sion of dementia fear and anxiety, we consider these emotions as experienced by persons who have received the diagnosis as well as persons who have not expe-rienced any obvious symptoms. In addition, we note how fear and anxiety rever-berate through the lives of those caring for loved ones who have dementia.

Psychological Perspectives on Fear and Anxiety

Although we typically think of fear and anxiety as negative emotions, they are actually neither positive nor negative. To understand the "valence" of an emotion,[3] we need to grasp the interaction between the person and the situation. Fear functions as an alarm system to protect creatures from danger. When frightened by some kind of threat, our nervous systems respond rapidly and organize behaviors of "fight or flight." Thus, in many situations, fear turns out to be positive because of its protective function. On the other hand, if we become paralyzed by fear and can neither defend ourselves nor flee, then fear is maladaptive and dangerous.

Fear is one of the first emotions infants experience. Although it will be many years before they can use words to describe subjective experience of fear, their cries and facial expressions clearly communicate their inner state. Certain actions automatically elicit fear responses from babies, which is the reason why strangers should not suddenly "loom" over them when they are happily sitting in their strollers.[4] Darwin (1872/1965) believed that the emotions that appear so early in life were selected through evolution to keep the young organism relatively free from danger. Most adults recognize and quickly respond to these fear behaviors, thus keeping the baby safe.

Anxiety, on the other hand, takes much longer to emerge as part of the human repertoire of emotion. Like fear, anxiety makes us want to hide to escape or avoid trouble. But, unlike fear, which is elicited by a sudden, definable, threatening situation, anxiety's source is more opaque or ambiguous. One way of thinking about this is that anxiety is experienced as anticipation that something bad is going to happen in the future, though its exact form is unclear. Fear is the response to a threat right now, in front of us.

Christine, who has had a diagnosis of Alzheimer's disease for about four years, described how she first realized she had a problem. "I found myself driving and forgetting where I was going. It scared the bejeebers out of me." She lives alone and decided she should seek help, so she went to her doctor, who sent her to a memory clinic where she had an MRI and a battery of neuropsychological tests. She has become very active in a local support group for people with the diagnosis and has enthusiastically embraced a new diet, with "lots of fruits and veggies and walnuts." She is proud of getting her blood pressure under control and lowering her cholesterol. Even though she lives in a part of the country with severe winters, she makes a point of walking outside nearly every day. She volunteers at her church, especially during the Green Bay Packers season, when she helps make and serve a northeast Wisconsin treat called "booyah" (a kind of stew) to raise money for church programs. Reflecting on her memory problems, her difficulty following conversations, and her bouts of confusion, she said, "I don't let it bother me, but sometimes it does. Mostly I don't give it a second thought."

Christine's fear motivated her to seek a diagnosis. In addition to her new diet, exercise program, and engagement with her support group and church, she takes medications typically prescribed for persons in the early stages of Alzheimer's disease, as well as drugs to control her blood pressure and cholesterol level. Her physician treats her as a collaborator in maintaining her health, giving her a sense of control. Thus, while her fear led her to a diagnosis, the diagnosis has turned out to be a positive experience because it has allowed her to make decisions that support her sense of well-being. Experiences like Christine's have been documented by researchers who study people's reactions when their physicians say they have a form of dementia. Although we might think that it would be devastating, in many cases people actually feel relief to finally have an explanation for their frightening experiences of forgetfulness and confusion (Carpenter 2009).

Though different, fear and anxiety are often connected in our experiences of threat. If we are unable to cope with a frightening situation, then, still aroused, we may feel the anxiety of not knowing what will happen next. This disturbs our sense of a world that is predictable and meaningful. Richard Lazarus, the psychologist whose work taught us much about stress and coping, said that "anxiety arises when existential meaning is disrupted or endangered" (1991, 234).

As forgetting increases and produces greater confusion, persons who have dementia are more apt to encounter frightening situations. Suddenly, the familiarity we expect in our worlds disappears. "Who are you? Why are you here? What are you doing to me?" These are the cries of the person who has dementia and cannot recognize familiar people and places. Calm replies and focusing attention on something familiar (a cozy chair, perhaps) may reduce the fear, but the anxiety about an unpredictable, crazy-meaningless world may persist. People who are living with dementia who can still describe their experiences talk about "strangeness" and a nagging sense of unreality. Another way that anxiety can be expressed is through suspiciousness. If I cannot recall what I did with my purse, then I may assume that someone stole it. And if someone is stealing my purse, what else might they take from me? The existential meaning offered by an orderly world in which we can exercise effective control can quickly disappear in the face of constant forgetting.

Care partners experience the fears and anxieties of those for whom they care as well as their own fears and anxieties. For example, imagine the fear of the daughter who kisses her father good-bye in the morning, goes to the grocery expecting that he will maintain his usual routine of watching game shows, and returns to find him missing. The fear may recede once her father is safely home again (perhaps brought by a police officer), but surely anxiety will remain. She does not know when this will happen again. Knowing her father was sitting in his favorite chair watching game shows used to be a predictable part of her life. Now it is not.

Like fear, which can motivate us to seek safety, anxiety can also be adaptive as long as it does not overwhelm our capacity to cope. For example, if students have mild to moderate levels of anxiety about an upcoming exam, they may be more motivated to study for it. On the other hand, if they experience no anxiety about the exam, they may not study at all, and if they have so much anxiety that their hearts race, their mouths are dry, they feel like they cannot breathe, and they cannot focus their attention, then studying for the exam becomes impossible.

The daughter whose father wandered might be able to transform her anxiety into action (perhaps by investing in a monitoring system), but if she is overwhelmed by the anxiety, she may not be able to make good decisions about his care or about taking good care of herself. A similar observation can be made about a perfectly healthy person who feels anxious about the possibility of developing dementia. These people are sometimes labeled the "worried well."[5] Their anxiety may motivate them to eat better, exercise more, turn off the mindless television shows, practice various cognitive fitness activities, and become involved in stimulating social groups. However, such positive life changes will elude the individual who minimizes warnings about heart health and brain health or whose anxiety is so great that despair and fatalism pervade everyday life.

People differ in how they respond to both specific and vague threats. These responses are shaped in part by a kind of biological thermostat, which regulates how the body reacts to threat and varies in sensitivity among persons. Psychologically, fear and anxiety can be woven into the fabric of personality. Some people describe themselves as "worry warts," more ready to feel anxious about unpredictable, uncertain events and vigilantly watchful for situations that might cause fear. Psychologists describe this as "trait anxiety," which is different from the "state anxiety" people feel from time to time when their sense of the world as meaningful and ordered is disturbed.

Sometimes, people experience fear and anxiety persistently and intensely; they feel overwhelmed and helpless to cope either with the perceived danger right in front of them or the anticipated threat. Clinically, we would say they have tipped into the psychopathology of phobia (undue fear about specific things), panic, or one of many other kinds of anxiety disorder (Öhman 2000). When fear and anxiety become unmanageable and maladaptive for care partners, persons with the diagnosis, or the "worried well," therapy should be sought. Although in our age, psychiatric problems are often treated only with medications (which in the case of anxiety and depression can be effective), attending support groups or having regular conversations with a skilled clinician can provide valuable guidance for coping with the threats and uncertainties that elicit fear and anxiety.

Terror Management

We told the story of Dorothy and Gardner in Chapter 3. Dorothy was doing her best to care for Gardner as his memory loss and confusion grew worse. Many of their friends were encouraging her to "place him" in some kind of memory-care residence. They thought that demonstrating friendship and support required them to urge her to devote more care to herself. They were probably right in some of their advice; she did need to take care of herself, but she needed to do so in order to continue to care for Gardner.

We do not in any way think those friends were bad people. On the contrary, they sound like many well-meaning people, and at least they were staying in contact with Dorothy. Other friends had drifted away, which is a scenario often reported by care partners.

We have seen that some psychological approaches to fear and anxiety are neutral on whether these are positive or negative responses to threats, and we noted that people have different ways of responding to experiencing these feelings. People make conscious choices about how they manage emotions (a topic we address again in the next chapter). This is the main idea of socioemotional selectivity theory, which we mentioned in the last chapter, when we described research showing that as people grow older, they choose to spend time in social situations that are more positive and less upsetting, aggravating, or confusing.

Some of Dorothy and Gardner's friends were coping with Gardner's situation by choosing to spend less time with Dorothy and Gardner. But, how were they making these choices? Perhaps they were saying this (either publicly or privately): "Gardner makes me anxious. I don't know how to deal with him anymore and seeing him like he is, makes me worry about whether I might be like that someday, too. I'm not going to call or visit Dorothy and Gardner because it's just too upsetting." Or, perhaps the friends *were* feeling anxious about being around Gardner and about their own unknown futures. However, rather than deliberately deciding not to call or visit, time just slipped by, they got busy and distracted, and they simply never got around to checking in with Dorothy and Gardner. When they spotted Dorothy and Gardner out for a walk, they always had some good reason to hurry on by, with just a wave and a shouted "hello."

Psychologists have begun to investigate whether anxiety about the unknown future motivates people to behave in ways that do not feel like conscious choices. In other words, is it possible that some of those friends of Dorothy and Gardner were unaware that they seemed to be avoiding them? According to a new subfield of social psychology called terror management theory (TMT),[6] those friends might have had no conscious sense of what was guiding their behavior.

Nearly all research on terror management focuses on the ways people behave when they are feeling fearful or anxious about death. Psychologists bring people into their laboratories and randomly assign them to one of two groups. One group will be asked to write a paragraph about death or to do some other kind of exercise involving death, such as matching words to pictures related to death. This is called priming. Supposedly the participants experience an activation of emotion as a result of the exercise, but they do not really notice the emotion, nor are they consciously aware of how that emotion might affect their subsequent behavior. Another group of participants will have a "pain prime," and write a paragraph about having a tooth drilled without a painkiller or match words and pictures related to pain. These exercises are called mortality salience inductions (although technically, only the one about death refers to mortality). After this, the participants are distracted for a little while, and then they are given some other kind of task. For example, they might complete a survey about their attitudes toward immigrants, terrorists, people who hold political values different from their own, or even people who have disabilities. They might also have their sense of self-esteem challenged or tested in some way.

When people are primed to feel anxious or fearful about death, they usually restrict their thinking to what the researchers call their cultural worldviews. In other words, they are less open to or tolerant of ideas that differ from their own or to people who are different from themselves. Similarly, people protect their sense of self-esteem—the notion that they are persons of value in a meaningful world—when they have been primed with emotions connected to death

(Solomon, Greenberg, and Pzszczynski 2004). They show this by choosing more positive attributes about themselves (e.g., offered in a fake horoscope or personality test result) after they have been reminded of their own mortality.

How does all of this connect to dementia? Research has shown that exposure to persons who have disabilities activates fears of death, and that when people are reminded of death (as in the kind of exercises we have described), they withdraw from people who live with disabilities. In other words, a person who has a disability threatens people's views of the world (everyone should be healthy and fit) and their self-esteem (my value comes from being healthy and fit) (Hirschberger, Florian, and Mikulincer 2005).

To test how this might apply to older adults, especially those who have memory loss, Susan and a graduate student had undergraduates read information describing either a young person or an older person who had just had a physical exam.[7] There were four outcomes: no information, normal results from three common medical tests, rheumatoid arthritis, or Alzheimer's disease (named *Gilson's disease* for the young adult, but having the same symptoms of progressive memory loss and disorientation). This produced eight possible descriptions. After completing several surveys on their feelings toward these eight pretend people, participants did a "word-stem completion task." This means that they were given parts of words and asked to complete them. For example, if they were given *r* and *i* and two blanks, they could write *rice* or *ring*. Some of the word stems, however, had the possibility of being completed with words connected to death. For example, *coff___* could either be *coffee* or *coffin*. We found significantly more death-related words produced by the participants who read about someone diagnosed with Alzheimer's disease. Obviously, much more research on this needs to be conducted, but our findings seem to be in line with those of others who have noted not only that disability is associated with death but also that old age in general activates people's anxieties about mortality (Martens, Goldenberg, and Greenberg 2005).

TMT researchers would not be surprised by stories like the one about Dorothy, Gardner, and their friends or by the many other anecdotal reports of friends withdrawing as dementia progresses. Perhaps these people are not consciously making the decision to fall out of friendship, but rather are reducing their dementia fear and anxiety (and possibly their fear and anxiety about death) while protecting their views of the world and their own sense of worth and value.

Social Sources and Consequences of Fear and Anxiety

So far, we have taken a largely psychological approach to fear and anxiety, but as we have repeatedly stated, people live in a social context. Because of the ways they motivate behavior, fear and anxiety are often cleverly manipulated in order to persuade people to purchase things or to donate money. For example, we recently received a plea for money from an organization that supposedly supports research on dementia and has a 31 percent (or, one star out of a possible four) ranking by www.charitynavigator.org. This reflects its high fundraising expenses compared to program expenses. The mailing came with a letter that urged us to send for a free pamphlet to learn more about "this mind-killer," also called "this sinister disease." Words like *horror, cruel,* and *victim* are repeated throughout the letter. A postscript repeats the warning that "Alzheimer's will strike again soon! There's not a minute to spare." A one-page statement about Alzheimer's disease enclosed with the letter says nothing about the persons and their families who live with it. All we learn is that these people are threatening to bankrupt the U.S. economy.

Many other examples of this kind of fear-mongering are documented in *Forget Memory* (Basting 2009). Once one becomes attuned to this kind of language, one begins to notice it more. A 2008 *New York Times* article about the "brain-fitness industry" talked about decaying brains (Hafner 2008). Humans and other animals have a built-in disgust response to decay and putrefaction (Rozin, Haidt, and McCauley 2000). Describing a living person's brain as decaying invites avoidance of that person. The same article quotes a person who works for a national aging group as saying that decline in brain function "is probably one of the most frightening aspects of the changes we undergo as we age." She continued by asserting that "our memories are who we are."

Social reinforcement of dementia dread is not a recent development. Rather, as so ably described by historian Jesse Ballenger (2006), it dates back to the nineteenth century, when a change occurred in how people constructed a sense of self. Rather than relying on social institutions like families and religions to create a structure for identity, each individual person was expected to do this alone. As compared to earlier times, when "senility" was viewed as a part of some people's aging—people who would continue to be held within the bonds of community and communal memory—the end of the nineteenth century brought a different view: when memory failed, the individual's scaffold of selfhood collapsed. The woman quoted as saying "our memories are who we are" articulated this new vision of selfhood well. Without memories, who are we? And if we no longer are a "self," then why should the community invest scarce resources to maintain the empty shell?

In his book, Ballenger weaves a tale of individual fears and anxieties stimulating governments and private organizations to fund research and policy initiatives that were then sustained by more dread experienced by more persons. The dread spread from individuals worried about their own futures to social institutions anticipating the "age wave." The image of the age wave burst on the national scene in 1990 when a 38-year-old psychologist/gerontologist named Ken Dychtwald published a book called *The Age Wave*. The book dealt with the demographics of the baby boom (persons born between 1946 and 1964) and projections that by 2030, one out of every five people in the United States would be 65 years old or older. By 2007, the age wave had morphed into a *tsunami*, a word used repeatedly at a national aging conference that year. Everyone knew that a real tsunami had struck in the Indian Ocean in 2004, killing more than 200,000 people. Thus, the connection was secured between an aging society and death and destruction.

The same year that Dychtwald's (1990) book appeared, a quieter article appeared in a rather obscure journal. There, Ann Robertson (1990) asserted that projections of burden to society by an aging population susceptible to Alzheimer's disease and other dementias amounted to "apocalyptic demography." Robertson carefully analyzed how old age was becoming biomedicalized, as it was increasingly defined as a problem that needed to be solved with medical interventions. With the development of more finely calibrated tools for measuring cognitive function—in terms of both brain imagery and mental testing—along with increasing public awareness of age demographics, the stage was set for a drama of tragedy and terror.[8]

This drama has consequences for persons who are living with dementia, their care partners, and the people (possibly friends) who are frightened and worried that they themselves might slip into progressive forgetfulness and confusion. To illustrate this, we describe three interviews: one with a person who is living with dementia and two with family members who accepted the primary responsibilities of caring for their loved ones.

Jane was diagnosed with early-stage dementia about a year after first noticing that she was forgetting what she had talked about in phone conversations with her daughter. Sitting in the cozy, sunny home that she now shares with her daughter, she talked about things that worry her (forgetting dates) and things that bring her joy (family, walking in her neighborhood, playing the piano).

Speaking of other people's reactions to her memory loss, she described uncomfortable interactions with a special friend who made fun of her for forgetting and was annoyed when she repeated herself in conversations. She also talked about shame and how people do not want to talk with her about her diagnosis. "They wouldn't mind asking me about having the flu," she said.

Holly sat at the farmhouse kitchen table with her father, Marv, who has lived with Alzheimer's for several years. Marv didn't talk much, but he smiled often and joked about his selective hearing. When the conversation turned to his work as a milk tanker driver, he became more talkative. Toys belonging to three young children were scattered about on the floor. In addition to Holly, her husband, her father, and children, three dogs, several cats, a cockatiel, and a lot of tropical fish live in this old farmhouse, the place where Holly had grown up. She and her family moved back into it to take care of her father. Holly tries to get as much information about dementia as she can, but she lives in a rural area, without high-speed Internet access, and few services are available to her and her father. When asked about whether she gets help from anyone, she said wistfully, "I'm sure there are people who want to help but they just don't know how to approach it. People don't call here much; they don't stop in as often."

For more than four years, Gloria has cared for her husband, George, who has frontotemporal dementia. She takes him to an adult day program three days a week, but she's not very happy with the type of care he gets. (Several months after our interview, the structure of the program changed its focus to younger people who have developmental disabilities, and her husband was asked to leave.) She said, "Our friends have kind of moved on from us. We're not really chummy with our neighbors. I just don't want to burden people with my troubles. My family will say a lot that they'll come down and be with him, but they rarely come. Our society can be too busy. People who have dementia are just wonderful people who have hit a bump in the road of their lives. I don't tell my kids everything that George does; otherwise they wouldn't talk to me."

These individuals, and many others with whom we spoke, seem to be resigned to the fact that people will make little effort to stay in touch with them once they or the ones they love cross the threshold of dementia. Perhaps they, too, have accepted the view of selfhood that says that once memory fades, there is little left to engage the interest or attention of anyone other than people willing to step forward and accept the responsibilities of being in a care partnership with someone traveling the dementia road. In effect, all these people are suffering what is sometimes called social death. The father of American psychology, William James, described it like this: "If no one turned round when we entered, answered when we spoke, or minded what we did, but if every person we met 'cut us dead,' and acted as if we were non-existing things, a kind of rage and impotent despair would ere long well up in us, from which the cruelest bodily tortures would be a relief; for these would make us feel that, however bad might be our plight, we had not sunk to such a depth as to be unworthy of attention at all" (1890/1950, 293–94).

It is possible that the people we interviewed felt this rage and despair at times but were too polite, or ashamed, to speak of it with us. James's description closely matches the way John Bowlby (1969–80) talked about children who felt abandoned by the people (usually parents) to whom they were emotionally attached. They responded first with protest and then with despair. James's image of being cut dead also reminds us of Kitwood's (1997) description of the malignant social environment that we described earlier. It helps us understand some of the challenging behaviors observed in people living in some institutional settings. These range from withdrawl to screaming and striking others.

Alzheimer's disease has been described as a "disease of exclusion" (Corner and Bond 2004, 153), and the same could be said for the other dementias. Why are people so reluctant to reach out to persons with the diagnosis and the courageous family members who care for them? Drew Christianson (1995), a Roman Catholic ethicist, suggests that they remind us of our two deepest anxieties about aging: that we will be abandoned and dependent on others. The issue of abandonment is fraught with contradiction, because out of anxiety over being abandoned, people abandon others. Abandonment is terrifying because of our biologically based need to be in relationship with others, especially those to whom we are emotionally attached.

Anxieties about dependency can often be managed by avoiding encounters with those who are dependent, which is, of course, ultimately a futile effort because all human beings are vulnerable and dependent on others, as we argued in Chapter 3 and earlier in this chapter. However, in our time, adults do develop temporarily effective strategies to avoid being reminded of dependency. Refusing to visit friends in hospitals and nursing homes is one common tactic.

One more focus of anxiety needs to be added to the two we have already named: identity and the threats posed by dementia. In his book on the history of senility in America, Ballenger shows how this anxiety grew through the twentieth century. People are anxious not only that loss of memory could mean loss of identity but also that the persons who have already experienced memory loss might have forgotten who they are. We want to be recognized by others, and when we are not, we experience a tinge of what William James described.

A common question asked of a spouse, son, daughter, or close friend of an individual who is living with dementia is "Does she [or he] know you?" Even if not asked, people quickly volunteer this information. For example, when Maria Shriver was interviewed about the four-part documentary she produced for HBO called *The Alzheimer's Project*, she responded to the question "How is your dad" (Sargent Shriver, who had AD) by saying, "He still looks terrific, but he doesn't know who I am." This intense concern about the preservation of identity in the memory of another person becomes even more problematic when it is directed at the person who has memory loss. As we remarked in Chapter 5, entering the room of a friend or relative and beginning the conversation by saying, "Do you know who I am?" is a guaranteed way of increasing the anxiety of everyone present.

Fear and anxiety about dementia create barriers to social contact that have the psychological effect of increasing the fear and anxiety of the person who elicited these feelings in the first place. These barriers also have biological consequences because they prevent social interactions, which can be good for overall health and well-being. More than a half-century of research has shown us that meaningful social connections support longevity and may even protect against the onset of progressive forgetfulness (see Fratiglioni, Paillard-Borg, and Winblad 2004). Having a larger social network also seems to be associated with less cognitive impairment, even when the plaques and tangles that indicate Alzheimer's disease are present (Bennett et al. 2006).

People often speak of the warmth of human contact and warm feelings between those who care for one another. Conversely, social exclusion literally makes people feel cold. An "icy stare" is not simply a figure of speech; it reflects physiological mechanisms demonstrated in a laboratory where people who were excluded from an activity, compared to those who were included, had a greater desire for warm food and drink and estimated the temperature of the room as being lower (Zhong and Leonardelli 2008). Moreover, the pain of social exclusion is real; hurt feelings produce pain that people remember better and more intensely than physical pain (Chen et al. 2008). Finally, the neural alarm system that signals social exclusion overlaps with the system used to signal physical pain (Eisenberger and Lieberman 2004; MacDonald and Leary 2005), an observation that has been made both in humans and in social animals.

All this reminds us of a statement we read in a book on the neuroscience of love: "A relationship *is* a physiologic process, as real and as potent as any pill or surgical procedure" (Lewis, Amini, and Lannon 2000, 81). This suggests the misguided focus in care that relies only on medications to treat Alzheimer's disease and other forms of dementias. Here is how George and Whitehouse put their tongues in their cheeks to talk about this idea: "Telling a story, reading a book, or participating in talk therapy engenders complex but undoubtedly real changes in the brain. In fact, it is not a stretch to refer to reading a book as a multineurotransmitter, neuroprotective, lexical access enhancement device, especially when pills tend to act on only one or just a few primary neurotransmitter systems!" (2009, 20). We prefer just to talk about reading, but we do appreciate the point George and Whitehouse are making.

CHAPTER SEVEN

Beyond Fear and Anxiety

The monologue continues:

> Yup! You've got it right: I'm scared and I'm worried about my forgetfulness. My friends all joke about it. But what good is it to know what psychologists say about fear and anxiety? I want to know what to do about it! Isn't there some kind of pill I could take?

For starters, our imaginary friend might read Anne Basting's (2009) book *Forget Memory*.[1] In the concluding chapter, Basting writes that we need to get beyond the fear so that we can create better lives for persons who are living with dementia and, in the process, create a better world for all persons to grow old in. Basting insists that people need to find the courage to ignore the sound bites of tragedy found in so many accounts of people who are living with dementia.

We do not deny that dementia brings painful loss to persons who have the diagnosis and to their families and friends, and we will say more about suffering in a later chapter. But, through the journey of dementia, there can also be growth and joy. Keeping these opposing images from flying apart poses a challenge to all of us, but if we are going to create communities where all persons are valued, regardless of their mental status, then we need to learn how to do this. Basting describes the kinds of advocacy activities that must occur to create communities where people are proud to acknowledge and take responsibility for their interdependency and where memory loss does not have to produce shame. She makes the important point that young people need and want to be a part of this effort. Contrary to stereotypes about their sense of entitlement, many young adults really do care about making a better world for people living with memory loss. This may come as a surprise to politicians and marketers whose simplistic parsing of generations leaves the impression that people care only about others in their own age group.

Basting's final point on her list of twelve ways to get beyond fear is worth quoting: "Don't be afraid of reducing fear" (2009, 165). She notes that perpetuating fear and anxiety about dementia helps organizations' fundraising, because fear may motivate people to donate money to support the search for a cure for the condition that elicits the fear. Some organizations may be afraid of eliminating the connection of this powerful aversive emotion to memory loss. But consider the implications of not reducing the fear. Try to imagine a world in which increasing numbers of persons receive the diagnosis of some form of dementia and have to learn to live not only with memory loss but also with the stigma, social malignancy, and excess disability that flourish in a fear-saturated environment.

We would rather imagine a different scenario, one in which people have the courage to acknowledge that progressive memory loss may come to any of us, that we are all traveling the dementia road together, and that we are not driving our own vehicles, isolated from one another and using up Earth's resources to preserve that isolation. The image of traveling this road together reminds us of a time when a new highway was built in our city, part of which included a bridge spanning a beautiful section of the river on which the city had been built more than 150 years earlier. Before the highway opened to vehicles, pedestrians were invited to explore it. People swarmed to see this new highway, especially the view of the river from the bridge. Parents pushed strollers and people propelled themselves in wheelchairs; some rode bicycles and others skimmed along on skateboards. It was a beautiful autumn day, and the shared joy of a huge group of people gathered where individuals in the privacy of their cars and trucks would soon be traveling at high speeds was palpable. In just a few days, people would be terrified to walk, run, skate, or wheel on this road, but for those few hours, there was no fear. There was community.

In the introduction to *Ageing, Disability, and Spirituality*, Elizabeth MacKinlay (2008a) relates a story of how fear drives people apart. After one of her public lectures, MacKinlay, an Anglican priest, geriatric nurse, and director of the Centre for Ageing and Pastoral Studies in Canberra, Australia, was approached by a person who wanted to know if it was all right to tell people who are living with dementia in nursing homes that one of their friends had died. It seems this individual was worried about protecting the privacy of the person who died. However, that concern for privacy was a mask, hiding the fear of confronting another person's grief. MacKinlay said, "If fear drives the agenda, then compassion is driven out. The need of vulnerable elderly people to know about their friends must be honoured. To deny the reality of life and death on the basis of 'privacy' is to move outside any compassionate understanding within society" (17).

Because she had also known fear, MacKinlay could be compassionate toward the person who posed the question to her. Elsewhere in her book, she describes her fear when Christine Bryden asked if she would be willing to be her spiritual adviser. Bryden, a 46-year-old mother of three young children, had recently been diagnosed with early-onset dementia.[2] MacKinlay said that her "biomedical model informed through years of nursing wanted to say 'no' to her request. I wanted to run, anywhere but into being so close to someone who had dementia" (2008b, 50). However, instead of running away, MacKinlay prayed. Only then could she agree to enter into that deep form of relationship that is spiritual care. With the support of MacKinlay, her husband, and many others, Bryden found the courage to reach out to people who have dementia through her public speaking and writing (Bryden and MacKinlay 2008). For her part, MacKinlay learned that the commitment she made to journey with Bryden enriched her life in multiple ways and inspired much of the work she currently does to help people move beyond dementia fear and anxiety.

MacKinlay said that fear can drive out compassion, but, quoting 1 John 4:18, "perfect love casts out fear." However, in reflecting on perfect love—God's love for creation—MacKinlay realized that human beings have imperfect love. Nevertheless, even imperfect love represents a major step beyond fear and anxiety. The challenge, of course, is that this is one of many things in life that is much easier said than done.

Peace and Love

Joseph de Rivera is a social psychologist who directs the Peace Studies Program at Clark University in Worcester, Massachusetts. It might seem odd to turn to the work of a person involved with peace studies to teach us about moving beyond dementia fear and anxiety to love and compassion. However, a paper de Rivera published in 1989 provides helpful guidance in thinking about this difficult subject. De Rivera began his essay like this: "We live in a new world of immense promise and difficulty. Our technological advances give us the means to feed, clothe, and shelter billions of new human beings, to prolong health, to offer immeasurable opportunities for adventure, pleasure, meaningful work—joy and serenity for all. Yet we have hunger, homelessness, torture and war" (387).

We would add that we also have loneliness and ostracism experienced by people whose brains developed plaques, tangles, and other pathological features of dementia earlier, more quickly, and more densely than the brains of the rest of us. Technological advances, particularly in the biomedical domain, have added years to life, but so far, no one has found a way to turn back the tide of progressive forgetfulness that so many older people live with. Wealth (even in a time of recession) has enabled for-profit and not-for-profit organizations to build and staff memory-care facilities, many of which are upscale. Nevertheless, people who have memory loss can live for weeks or more without contact with anyone but people paid to care for them. Although these care providers may be skilled, loving, and compassionate, many "facilities" still seem like small fortresses surrounded by moats in cities and towns across America. And, as we have noted repeatedly, it is not just people in long-term care residences who are isolated; individuals living with the effects of the early stages of progressive forgetfulness also suffer exclusion, as do their care partners.

To explain how a peace psychologist can guide us through the thicket of worry and fright about forgetfulness, we need to take a brief detour through two books by John Macmurray (1957, 1961), a Scottish philosopher, whose work has been a major influence not only on de Rivera's work but also on the writings of another Scot, John Swinton. In his many books and articles, Swinton presents a model of personhood that applies to people living with various intellectual and mental health problems, including those diagnosed with schizophrenia and bipolar disorder (2000), developmental disability (2008), learning disability (Swinton and McIntosh 2000), and, of course, dementia (2007).

John Macmurray's Gifford Lectures

In 1953 and 1954, John Macmurray, professor of moral philosophy at the University of Edinburgh, delivered a series of lectures at the University of Glasgow. Macmurray thus took his place in a long line of distinguished scholars invited to present the Gifford lectures. Begun in 1888 with a bequest from Adam Lord Gifford to four Scottish universities,[3] the Gifford lecture series has been offered continuously with the exception of the war years 1942–45. The general topic of the lecture series, as directed by Lord Gifford, is to be "natural religion," that is, a consideration of religion apart from the mysteries of revelation.

Being asked to prepare and give these lectures is generally regarded as one of the greatest honors a scholar in philosophy, science, or religion can receive. The list of luminaries who have been Gifford scholars attests to this. Best known among psychologists is the series of lectures given in 1900–1901 by William James, and later published as *The Varieties of Religious Experience*. It is difficult to name just a few of the other distinguished Gifford scholars, but using the criterion of name recognition for some and noting that the ideas of others, perhaps less well known, have been referenced in this book, we offer this partial list, ordered according to when they presented their lectures: Alfred North Whitehead, Albert Schweitzer, Karl Barth, Reinhold Niebuhr, Niels Bohr, Paul Tillich,

Hannah Arendt, Iris Murdock, Carl Sagan, Alisdair Macintyre, Martha Nussbaum, and Stanley Hauerwas.

In Macmurray's first series of lectures, published as *The Self as Agent* (1957), Macmurray argued that we need to think about a self as a doer and not as a thinker. The image of the self as a thinker has dominated Western philosophy and psychology (with the exception of the behaviorists, who emphasized the doing but saw no need to talk about "the self"). This doing, which Macmurray linked to the essence of selfhood, is not merely an automatic response to a stimulus; rather, it is the result of intentional initiation of action.

Can people who have dementia do this? Can they intentionally initiate action? Macmurray's aim was to do philosophy, not to meditate on the selfhood of people who have cognitive impairments. However, he prompts us to pose these questions and to observe that the answers are "yes" across the spectrum of dementia. Most individuals experiencing the early stages of memory loss still live independently.[4] They drive, shop, cook meals, entertain friends, make love, garden, dance, play, work. All of these actions reflect intent. But what about the person who has had to relocate to a nursing home, the person who may have lost all or nearly all language ability, who needs help engaging in the common activities of daily living?[5] By viewing their selfhood in terms of doing, not thinking, we can see that they, too, demonstrate the kind of selfhood in action that Macmurray describes. Here is an example from a study using observations made at a memory care residence: "Marge gets off the couch and starts touching objects in the living room. She throws a rag on the desk, takes her plate to the sink. She stops on her way to talk with Mary [another resident]. She says to a staff member, 'Are you sure you can take my plate?' She sees a knife on the counter and says, 'Shouldn't have a knife in the kitchen!' She will not give it to anyone; instead she insists on bringing it to the sink herself. 'I'm glad I caught this,' she says" (McFadden, Ingram, and Baldauf 2000, 75).

Note all the actions in this description and note also the interactions Marge has with other people. In the opening pages of the second book of Gifford lectures, *Persons in Relation*, Macmurray related that he had to use the first half of the lecture series to establish the idea of the self as doer, not as thinker or knower, to lay the groundwork for the second half of the series. In this book, he argued that "the Self is constituted by its relation to the Other; that it has its being in its relationship; and that this relationship is necessarily personal" (1961, 17). Later in the book, Macmurray distinguished between society and community, arguing that the former describes an impersonal bond among persons but that the connections in community are personal. This led him to differentiate between associates and friends, the former having relationships with others that serve themselves only (much like Aristotle's ideas of friendships of utility and pleasure) without the mutuality of caring for one another.

Capturing a brief glimpse of an ordinary moment in Marge's current life supports Macmurray's contention that we are constituted as selves in relation to others. Marge's statement, "I'm glad I caught this," implies that she is glad she caught the situation of the knife being placed somewhere she thought it did not belong for the sake of the safety of the others in the room. Marge cannot reflect philosophically on her sense of her selfhood as constituted through living in relationship with others, but she reveals it through her actions (including her utterance about the knife).

Macmurray's position on "persons in relation" reminds of us Tom Kitwood's (1997) definition of personhood and the efforts being made in many settings to transform the culture of dementia care by incorporating Kitwood's vision of persons living in relationship with one another. The old culture emphasizes loss and disability. An old culture interpretation of Marge would be of a woman with a brain mangled by tangles and plaques, rendering her incapable of autonomy, and making her needy and dependent. Yes, Marge has severe memory loss and so much confusion that she can no longer live alone. Nevertheless, she still is able to demonstrate agency—intentional interaction with her environment— and she bustles about the kitchen area of her communal residence, chatting with other persons, insisting on her own way of bringing order to the world and securing safety for others by placing the knife where it belongs, perhaps just as she once worked to maintain order in the kitchen of her own home.[6]

This chapter is about moving beyond fear and anxiety about dementia—fear and anxiety that keep us from interacting with persons living with forgetfulness— to love and compassion. However, as we show later, people cannot entirely let go of fear and anxiety. Seeing Marge wander about the kitchen area with the knife (which, by the way, was a table knife, not a sharp carving knife) might be a bit frightening, not because she might suddenly go on a knife-wielding rampage, but because she is a person who has dementia whose comments about the situation are somewhat unusual. Yet, if we are going to remain in friendship with persons like Marge, or even if we are going to consider the possibility of *becoming* friends with persons like Marge, then we need to learn how to see her and her actions in a new way, a way not shaped by fear for ourselves but motivated by love for the other. Macmurray elaborated on this difference in *Persons in Relation*. He said that a negative personal relationship—a relationship defined by fear, dislike, or mistrust—"makes knowledge of the other and of oneself alike impossible" (1961, 170).[7] When we fear for only ourselves, we are concerned with our own needs and whether they will be met, a position that reminds us of persons we described in Chapter 3 who experience insecure attachments to other persons.

The "Third Self": When Love Is More Powerful Than Fear

We now return to Joseph de Rivera's paper about love, fear, and justice. Although de Rivera made no reference to dementia, a close reading of his paper provides a way of thinking about the meaning of friendships with persons who are experiencing memory loss. De Rivera drew on Macmurray's Gifford lectures to formulate a position stating that neither individualism nor collectivism by itself can move the world toward peace and love. Rather, these two tendencies (expressed in individual lives as the tension between separateness and affiliation—or intimacy—with others) can complement each other. De Rivera's aim in this paper is to show how subordination of fear for the self frees people to care for others so that they can develop political systems that truly guarantee "justice for all." However, he also recognizes that his argument about selfhood—finding a "third way" alternative to the individualistic models of Western cultures and the collectivist models of Eastern cultures—can also apply to persons' lives as they are enacted on local stages.

The first step we need to take in understanding de Rivera's argument about the need to move to a position in which fear is subordinated to love is to examine what he means by *fear* and *love*. These terms are usually used to describe felt emotions, but de Rivera, who embraces Macmurray's ideas about the self as doer, argues that they should be taken more broadly to describe motivational forces that direct action. He described love as the "underlying motivational concern for the other" (1989, 402) and fear as the "underlying motivational concern for the self" (402). Interestingly, he says that the *emotions* (feelings) of fear and love can appear in the service of either fear or love, considered as motivational forces. To explain this, he writes:

> For example, one may feel the emotion of fear as one goes to help another out of love, or feel an emotion of love when one is really afraid of being alone. . . . Thus, behavior may be primarily oriented toward our concern/fear for ourselves or our caring/love for the other. However, the other motivational strand will also necessarily be present. Though subordinated, it will be contained within the action,

providing a complementary motivation. For example, when love is dominant, the subordinated fear is present in the maintenance of the boundary that preserves self-differentiation, or in realistic concerns for the safety of the other. (402)

The everyday lives of dementia care partners exemplify de Rivera's argument about the connection between fear and love. In the previous chapter, we briefly described Holly, who has been caring for her father, Marv, in the family farmhouse. Most of the time, she manages her complex life with calm and grace, but one night, when she got up and could not find him in his room, she was terrified. Her fear was amplified by her love. All care partners can identify with Holly's fear that night. At other, more ordinary times, when faced with the competing demands of her children, husband, and father, she feels the twinges of "subordinated fear"—concern for the self—as she wonders what would happen if she lost herself entirely in the care for others. What if she became so exhausted or stressed that she got ill? Would she still be able to care for her multigenerational family?

De Rivera writes that there are two different manifestations of the dominance of fear for the self over love for the other. He calls these "models of the self" (405), which he later contrasts with another model, which he names "the third self." In the first model, people become so concerned about maintaining boundaries between themselves and others that they cannot trust others. Fortunately, Holly does not fall into this category. She knows that when she has had a particularly challenging day, she can call her sister and vent to her. She trusts her sister's love and is secure enough to reveal her weaknesses to her.

Holly also avoids the second model of the self, in which fear for the self dominates concern for the other: mistrust of the worth of the self, which leads to "submissive conformism and lack of individuality" (404).[8] An example of how she does not follow this model can be found in the way she uses books she gets from her local library about her father's multiple medical problems, which make caring for him so complicated. She knows there is a lot of conflicting advice. Despite her lack of higher education, she is confident that she can make good decisions about the best use of advice from experts.

It is not hard to find examples of the motivational forces of fear and love in persons caring for loved ones who are living with dementia. But what about those not giving this kind of care, the friends to whom this book is primarily addressed? In earlier chapters, we described many sources of dementia fear and anxiety and the ways they lead to malignant social psychology, producing excess disability in those who live with the diagnosis. We can now see that in

light of de Rivera's two models of the self motivated by fear, a malignant social psychology results primarily from the first form, which builds walls between the self and the other. It is driven by people's desire for autonomy and
independence.

Related to the fear of memory loss is fear of the loss of independence.[9] People
who experience such fear avoid others who remind them of that possibility. They
may also fear that their cognitive capacity will be sullied through contact with
the person who has memory loss (i.e., they do not trust that they can be in relationship without losing part of themselves). This is expressed when people say,
"I can't go visit my friend, Joyce, because she just repeats herself over and over,
and says things that don't make sense, and by the time I've spent ten minutes
with her, I start to think I've got dementia, too!"

Sometimes, this type of fear for the self is rationalized by being transformed
into anxious concern that one's own life without dementia might make the person who has memory loss "feel bad." In other words, a person might say, "I can't
go visit my friend, Herb, because all I'd have to talk about would be my good,
rich, interesting life. Since he's had to move into a nursing home, seeing me will
make him feel worse about his situation."

These fears are understandable. No one wants to spend years in old age coping with progressive forgetfulness. As de Rivera says, "It would be unrealistic to
have no concerns for the self" (405). However, he does state that we need to learn
to subordinate (not eliminate) fear for the self to concern for the other; this is his
third model of the self. It stands in contrast with the two that are dominated by
fear. How might this third model look in terms of friends journeying with one
another through old age, knowing that some will undoubtedly experience memory loss? De Rivera describes seven outcomes that accrue when concern for the
other person dominates fear for the self.

First, people whose concern for others overrides their fear for themselves do
not need to worry that others will fail to meet their needs, or even that others
might not like them. The boundaries of the self are opened to permit mutuality—
a sense of "we" in which gains and losses are shared. Of course, this position
makes people vulnerable to the state of others. Time spent with a friend on the
dementia road will not always be pleasant and happy. It is hard to reach out to a
friend in grief, and even harder when that friend has memory problems and may
no longer be able to communicate in words. Nonetheless, as we have said from
the beginning of this book, time with our friends who have dementia can be
joyful. We offer some concrete suggestions on how to make it so in Chapter 11.
As we note there, as long as friends are sensitive to the changed experience of

other people and the environment that comes with progressive memory loss, many things can be mutually enjoyed and celebrated.

De Rivera states that a second gift of living with a ratio that favors concern for others over fear for the self lies in the lack of judgment of the other person's behavior. He does not say this facilely, nor does he imply that it is easy to get to the point of genuine acceptance in a relationship. Sometimes crossing this line and leaving judgment behind occurs when we can accept the changed appearance and behavior of another person. In the 1994 documentary film *Complaints of a Dutiful Daughter*, the filmmaker, Deborah Hoffmann, whose mother lives with dementia, describes how her mother always took pride in how she looked and acted. Her highly educated mother was not vain, but she was dignified and sophisticated in how she presented herself to the world both in behavior and in appearance. Thus, it was a shock to Debbie (as she is called in the film, by her mother), when she visited her mother at a memory-care residence after making the difficult decision that her mother needed full-time care and supervision. Her mother was wearing a light blue sweat suit and was happily singing an old-timey popular song, neither of which Debbie could have imagined her doing before the onset of forgetfulness. Debbie quickly recovered and celebrated the fact that her mother was happy and contented.

This leads us to de Rivera's next point: by containing fear, one can be fully in the moment with another person. After getting over her surprise about how her mother looked and was acting, Debbie joined right in, laughing and singing with her mother and the group of other old people who had dementia. People who have been friends for many years with someone who now cannot remember much and who has trouble ordering the world might also react as Debbie initially did to her mother's appearance and behavior. Having always known a friend to care about fashion and now seeing her padding about in a shapeless sweat suit would produce surprise. But, if concern for the friend dominates, then the two are freed to connect just as they are, with no pretense or judgment.

De Rivera's fourth observation about what happens when people allow their love to dominate over their fear is also illustrated in *Complaints of a Dutiful Daughter*: people can grow and discover new strengths through care for others that is not primarily motivated by fear. For a long time, before she realized her mother could no longer live alone, Debbie worked valiantly to control her mother's life. She thought she was demonstrating her love by securing her mother's independence. Thus, she meticulously wrote notes about appointments, talked by phone with her mother several times a day, managed her mother's finances, and undertook myriad other tasks, trying to hold her mother's life together. All this frantic activity was motivated by fear dominating love. When Debbie finally realized that her own fear was preventing her from accepting her mother's need for residential care, she experienced a deep sense of personal growth. Once she accepted her mother's need to move into a long-term care residence, she was freed to experience even deeper love for her mother.

De Rivera's fifth point notes how people can create solutions to problems that "benefit both parties" (406). This is of critical importance when relating to persons who have memory loss because most of them retain the ability to sniff out pretense and false conviviality. While we may be able to see the benefit of authentic friendship interactions that affirm the identity and value of the person who is living with dementia—interactions that produce joy and overcome loneliness—determining the benefit to the friend without progressive forgetfulness may require reflection on what can be learned from genuine moments of connection with someone whose condition so easily evokes fear and anxiety. In other words, there is much to be learned from critical self-reflection on one's motivation for spending time with a friend. Is it done because of a feeling of obligation or the need to do something that will be seen by others as righteous, or it is done because of the realization that spending time with a friend who has dementia can be beneficial to both persons? The answer to this question points to de Rivera's next observation: allowing love to be dominant frees people to be responsible and honest with one another. All people experience times when they would rather not relate to any other person—be it a friend who has dementia, a beloved child, an interesting neighbor, or a life partner—because of physical or psychological distress. Sometimes a person just wants to be alone, but if love and not fear is dominant in the relationship, the person requesting time alone knows that this need will pass and that the concern for the other endures.

De Rivera describes his seventh attribute of the "third model of the self" in this manner: "The person is able to move back and forth between what is ideal and what is real" (406). Debbie did not want her mother to have the diagnosis of Alzheimer's disease. She had imagined always having a mother who recognized her, remembered their history together, and could engage in lively discussion about Debbie's vocation and interests. She would never have wished this life for her or her mother. However, once she could accept what Freud called "the verdict of reality" (1917/1957, 255), she was set free to grieve the passing of one image of the ideal to realize another one, in which the ideal became the loving connection in the moment of contact with her mother, including the times when her mother was not sure of who she was or was confused about the nature of their relationship. "Did we go to school together?" her mother once asked her.

Being in friendship with a person who has dementia may require the reformulation of ideals about the relationship. Whereas we usually expect our friends to know us, remember the ways we have connected in the past, and be able to anticipate a future of meaningful interactions, our friend living with memory loss may not be capable of any of this. Thus, a new ideal must be embraced, one that seeks meaning in the experiences people share in the present moment. In other words, instead of saying "my friend has dementia, and I'm realistic about the fact that he can no longer really be a friend," one might say, "we had a good visit today, and I felt I received a gift by entering into the moment of just being together and not being occupied with the sundry details and pressures of day-to-day life." In other words, a new ideal has been created.

This ideal is challenging and may not be embraced by everyone all the time. Some will reject it outright, as threatening to weaken society by valuing relationships with persons who no longer can function independently as autonomous agents. Likewise, de Rivera's proposal that the "third self" model can move societies toward peace and justice would likely be greeted with derision by some people in our society. As philosopher Martha Nussbaum noted in her own Gifford lectures, delivered at the University of Edinburgh in 1992–93, "compassion is controversial. For about twenty-five hundred years it has found both ardent defenders, who consider it to be the bedrock of the ethical life, and equally determined opponents, who denounce it as 'irrational' and a bad guide to action" (2001, 354).

Everyone has days when he or she cannot or does not want to connect with others. No human being can experience perfect love; there will always be a measure of fear and anxiety about relationships, regardless of the other person's cognitive fitness. To be human is to live always with tension between attachment and detachment, between longing for meaningful connections with others and the desire for autonomous agency (Payne and McFadden 1994). Learning how to extract creative possibility from these two poles of human existence can liberate us to be whole persons living in flourishing communities that embrace and nurture persons with varying gifts and challenges.

To move beyond the kind of fear and anxiety that isolates and stigmatizes persons who are living with dementia and the ones who care for them, we need to start thinking about how we might form communities in which persons can support one another in the difficult task of subordinating fear for the self to love for the other. This will be challenging, but the alternative is a society that excludes persons who have memory loss. As de Rivera says, "mutuality is easier to conceive than to achieve" (410), and he was not even thinking about mutuality in relationships in which one or more persons lives with dementia.

In the next two chapters, we describe the contours of a flourishing community and suggest that support for relationships with friends who have dementia can be found in religious congregations, where people presumably hear frequent calls to love and compassion. We have no illusions, however, that religious beliefs and practices will necessarily tip the scale in favor of love for the other. De Rivera pointedly noted that the history of religion shows that it can support the two fear strategies (dominant individualism, which has the illusion of independence and control, or submissive conformism, which yields to powerful others) as well as the "third self" approach of subordinating fear to love. He wrote:

> One can pray in an attempt to control what happens in the real world; or one can pray to be accepted into an ideal heaven where justice will ultimately be rewarded; or one can pray for the capacity to forgive and the strength to aid the establishment of heaven on earth. In the first two, fear-motivated strategies, 'faith' means a sort of fear-motivated *belief*. In the third, faith means an *openness* to experience, a knowledge of one's ultimate worth, an acceptance of some Otherness that cannot be controlled and yet somehow helps things grow. (423)

Following our discussion of communities in general and congregational communities in particular, we return to the subject of faith. To de Rivera's description of the openness, knowledge, and acceptance inherent in faith, we add the notion of practices and examine how practices of love and friendship can sustain hope, even in the midst of suffering and loss.

CHAPTER EIGHT

The Flourishing Community

When we moved from the East Coast to the upper Midwest nearly thirty years ago, John was initially puzzled by some of the practices associated with weddings in this region. The couples planning their wedding were typically casual about the guest list. In a few cases their invitation took the form of a notice in the local newspaper. It was not uncommon for the wedding ceremony and the reception to be separated by four hours or more, almost as if they were unrelated events. Often the number of guests at the reception would be five times greater than those attending the wedding ceremony, which struck him as a profound discourtesy to the bride and groom.

An older Roman Catholic priest explained the origins of these local practices by noting that the region's roots lay in the small farming villages of northern Europe. In such villages, everyone was invited to a wedding because their lives had been deeply interwoven for generations. Because many of the guests were farmers, the wedding ceremony took place after the morning chores had been done and the reception occurred in the evening after the livestock had been fed, milked, and bedded down. And as for the social acceptability of attending the reception but not the ceremony, he explained with a twinkle in his eye, "Try to imagine a stubborn German farmer getting dressed in his best clothes twice on the same day!"

Those puzzling local wedding practices have largely vanished in the intervening decades. As is true elsewhere in our increasingly mobile society, most wedding guests now travel significant distances to participate in the festivities. They represent the many communities in which the bride and groom have participated in the course of their lives—families, friends from high school, friends from college, friends from their respective workplaces—rather than a single community in which the bride and groom were raised and will continue to live as a married couple.

For most of human history, community was something that was simply there, like the air around us. From the distinguished citizens (the banker, the priest or rabbi, the lawyer) to the village idiot, all shared in the fabric of common community, interacting with one another on a near-daily basis. If a community member's house burned, the community could be relied on to rally in support. If someone suffered serious illness, friends and neighbors would bring meals or assist in caring for children. And if an older member of the community journeyed into dementia, the community would adjust itself to the changes while continuing to incorporate that person into its common life.

It is not our intention to overly romanticize a bygone era or to discount the distinctions of class and race that created divisions in such communities, but merely to note that the concept of "self-selected community" is new in historical terms, largely driven by the explosion in mobility in the years following World War II. We recently spoke with a friend in her late sixties, a woman who enjoys a full and active postretirement life. She has two grown children, neither of whom lives in this area. Many of her closest friends have moved to other parts of the country to be closer to their children and grandchildren. Most of her remaining friends are fellow members of her church, but each Sunday she recognizes fewer of the faces around her. She can count on the fingers of one hand the number of persons living nearby whom she regards as close friends. "One of the things I worry about," she reflected, "is who I could ask to drive me home from the hospital if I needed surgery." Like many other people in our time, she draws a distinction between close friends, to whom she can comfortably turn in time of need, casual friends, on whom she is unwilling to impose, and a larger community—in this case, her church—to which she feels a meaningful connection but of which she has no personal expectations.

Community is a word that is bandied about in so many ways that its definition has become blurry. Even the audience that watches the same television program is referred to as a "community." But do we have a relationship with another person simply because he or she watches the same television program or owns the same consumer goods that we do?

Is Community a Fad, a Liberal/Conservative Conspiracy, or Something More?

In 1996, political scientist and journalist Fareed Zakaria wrote a "devil's dictionary" for what he described as the "intellectual buzzword of the '90s": *communitarianism*. Ideas about community, civil society, social capital, and civic engagement had become part of common political discourse, which naturally produced political controversy.[1] For example, Hillary Clinton, ever a magnet for strongly opposed positions, wrote a book called *It Takes a Village*, arguing that all people needed to be invested in the welfare of children in their communities.

Zakaria's "dictionary" had only three entries: *A* for Aristotle (who argued that humans are inherently political), *B* for bowling (referring to Robert Putnam's

book, *Bowling Alone*), and C for *civil society,* a term that describes vibrant voluntary organizations to some people, but for others is shorthand for political or
religious oppression. Zakaria noted that communitarianism was supposed to
offer a "third way," between liberal and conservative ideologies, but he said it had
become a meaningless word, ridden with political implications and despised by
many in both liberal and conservative camps.

The polarization of the late 1990s has not abated; in fact, it appears that the
opposing positions have grown even more entrenched. As noted by Putnam and
Feldstein, social capital—"social networks, norms of reciprocity, mutual assistance, and trustworthiness" (2003, 2)—can be used for good or for ill, by con-
servatives and liberals alike. Their book, *Better Together,* documents "best practices" in the United States, practices they believe strengthen communities and
improve the lives of the people who live in them. They make an important distinction between activities of *bonding,* in which like-minded people help one
another, and activities of *bridging,* when people who do not necessarily agree on
all things nevertheless put aside differences to create improvements in their
shared lives that benefit all. Obviously, the latter is much more challenging than
the former, especially in the context of extreme political polarization.

Research that attempts to address some of the questions raised in the debate
over communitarianism has examined changes in the size and makeup of
Americans' social networks. A nationally representative study comparing information gathered in 1985 and 2004 about whether people have others with whom
they can discuss important matters found a significant drop in the number of
confidants people have (McPherson, Smith-Lovin, and Brashears 2006). The
most frequent answer offered to the question "how many confidants do you have?"
was none in 2004; back in 1985, the most common answer was three. Although
the researchers did not ask specifically about whether people still bowled in
leagues, they did find that, overall, people had fewer contacts with voluntary
organizations and people in their neighborhoods in 2004 than they had had
in 1985.

Between 1985 and 2004, the term 24/7 entered the worldwide lexicon, driven
largely by technology that enabled people to work around the clock. Some might
argue that this technology also offered the opportunity to stay connected to people and that even if "face time" exchanges dropped, digital contacts increased.
We still have no clear understanding of whether Internet social networking provides the same kind of support for the human need to be connected with other
people.

Interestingly, hidden among all the statistics about Americans' shrinking social networks, there is one finding in the McPherson, Smith-Lovin, and Brashears (2006) study that offers a different picture. After slicing up their large sample by sex, education, race, and age, the researchers found shrinkage of social connections in nearly all categories with one exception: "the elderly have been more stable than most other groups in their core social connections" (371). The authors offer no explanation for this, though we might speculate that, despite the greater chance that they will experience the deaths of people in their "social convoys," older people have still clung to important rituals of friendship and community. As we show in the next chapter, one way they have traditionally done this is through their involvement in faith communities, where they have been encouraged to "bear one another's burdens" (Gal. 6:2).

Mutual Obligation

Community cannot exist without mutual obligation. We speak, for example, of the global community or the community of nations, recognizing not only that our lives are politically and economically interconnected but also that we have real obligations to one another (beginning with keeping the planet we share habitable). Indeed, harkening back to our definition of personhood in Chapter 3, if to be a person is to be vulnerable and dependent on others, then community can be defined as a web of relationships of mutual dependence and obligation among vulnerable persons.

For each of us, life begins in complete dependence. We rely on our parents for food, shelter, and protection. We require a community of responsible adults— parents, relatives, and teachers—to help us develop the knowledge and skills necessary to function in the world. We depend on others to care for us when we are ill, to comfort us when we are frightened, and to correct us when our behavior threatens our own or others' safety or well-being. The community around us nurtures, protects, shapes, and forms us as persons. One of the moral teachings we learn from the community is that from birth we are indebted to others and are required to reciprocate. We are schooled in the ways of gratitude and taught to express that gratitude by offering our help to those who need us.

Although our dependence on others may lessen as we move into adulthood, it remains at the core of our personhood. We turn to a former teacher to provide a recommendation for a college or a family friend to serve as a reference for a job application. An injury or illness may be suffered at any time, forcing us to depend on the care of others. We depend on police officers to protect our streets, firefighters to protect our homes, and various governmental entities to deliver our mail, maintain the peace, and secure justice. Even those institutions we are wont to complain about provide services and protections essential to our lives. We depend on friends and neighbors to give joy to our days, meaning to our lives, and a structure of norms and expectations that provide order and coherence in which our individual and corporate lives may flourish.

Our obligation to reciprocate can never be expressed in a tidy, symmetrical manner. The needs of a healthy child born to affluent, educated, high-functioning parents will be different from the needs of a child born with a disability or a child raised in extreme poverty. If we are that first, fortunate child, do our obligations extend only to our own parents and the specific individuals who contributed to our personal development? If we are the second, less fortunate child, can our parents and immediate family alone provide for all of our legitimate needs? What can we return to our parents proportionate to what they have given to us? If we tallied favors received and obligations incurred as if were dividing the bill from a restaurant meal, offering help and support only to those we personally "owed," the structure of community around us would quickly collapse.

Living in community, we participate in a complex network of relationships in which we both give and receive. If that community and the individual members of it (including ourselves) are to flourish, our giving and receiving will be based on our varying needs and abilities rather than "tit for tat" repaying of obligations to the specific persons who have helped us in the past. As expressed by Alasdair MacIntyre, "I have to understand that what I am called upon to give may be quite disproportionate to what I have received and that those to whom I am called upon to give may well be those from whom I shall receive nothing. And I also have to understand that the care I give to others has to be in an important way unconditional, since the measure of what is required of me is determined in key part, even if not only, by their needs" (1999, 108).

MacIntyre, senior research fellow in the Center for Ethics and Culture at the University of Notre Dame, argues the importance of "virtue ethics," which are centered in the habits and practices that help people understand how to share in a good life with others. It is his conviction that the effort to practice "the virtues" results in the formation of moral character, which in turn enables people to make good judgments. The goal of good judgments is to make decisions that allow the individuals who make them, as well as others, to flourish—to grow, thrive, and prosper—in a given environment or stage of development. MacIntyre argues that there is no condition or circumstance that makes flourishing impossible given the context of a community of persons committed to living lives of virtue. Reynolds (2008) further expands on what it means to flourish: "the prospering of an inbuilt human capacity to experience and share with others the multifaceted joy of being alive" (104).

Without a commitment to the common good and the conviction that every person's life has dignity, value, and worth, there can be no such thing as a flourishing community. The morality of a community, whether a nation-state or a local neighborhood, is measured by the care extended to its most vulnerable and dependent members. An individual life can flourish only in the context of a flourishing community, a community that seeks to honor, value, and include in its common life all of its members, particularly those who are most vulnerable and therefore in need of hospitality and friendship from others.

Sadly, virtually all communities are guilty of ostracizing those perceived to present a threat to the norms of the community. In some circumstances this is necessary and appropriate, as when a violent individual poses a legitimate threat to the safety of others or when a person who has a contagious disease must be quarantined. But in many cases persons are ostracized because they are perceived as not fitting in or because they embody truths that others do not wish to confront.

Ostracism is highly aversive because human beings are social creatures.[2] Some authors have suggested that while it is always painful to be excluded, most people would prefer punitive ostracism over "oblivious ostracism" because at least with the former, the person knows why the community has cast its attention away (Case and Williams 2004). If you are not considered worthy of attention at all—if people are oblivious to you, as Ralph Ellison so eloquently portrayed in his book *Invisible Man*—then you are treated as if you had already died. Such is the fate of some persons who have dementia.

It was not so many years ago that persons living with certain disabilities were routinely institutionalized not because their needs could be better met in such a setting but because their appearance might be "upsetting to children" or their presence disruptive to common life. They were guilty of reminding us of our own vulnerability and were therefore removed from sight. Their absence reduced the richness and honesty of the community, depriving its members of the opportunity to offer their gifts of support and friendship. Persons who have mental illness are still too often the victims of such stigmatization, as are persons who have been incarcerated.

Perhaps even more widespread is the practice of self-imposed withdrawal from community by those who perceive themselves as no longer having value to offer others. In a previous chapter we mentioned that a mere two decades ago the word *cancer* was spoken in hushed terms, and those who suffered from it felt the need to absent themselves from public life. The changes and losses that accompany aging can lead to similar withdrawal from the fabric of common life, often expressed through words like "I'm no good to anybody anymore" or "I don't want to be a bother to anyone." Pride often lies behind such sentiments. Gladys is embarrassed to be seen in a wheelchair. Arnold is terrified that he might suffer "a little accident" in public. Vulnerability is seen as shameful, rather than as the essential glue that defines relationships in a flourishing community.

In no case is this truer than when aging includes the journey into dementia. Rather than understanding dementia as an experience shared by the entire community, whose role and responsibility is to accompany a valued member on this journey, it is treated as a private tragedy to be dealt with by the individual, his or her family, medical professionals, and professional caregivers. To be sure, when certain dementias move into an advanced stage, care in a special treatment facility becomes necessary and unavoidable. Providing such facilities and ensuring that not just the quality of care but the quality of life within them allow individuals to flourish is one of the ways in which a community fulfills its obligation to the vulnerable (always mindful that we are equally vulnerable and may one day require such care).

Persons who have dementia who are still capable of participating in the life of the community outside of institutional care are too often permitted to withdraw from common life (sometimes at the insistence of family members who are suffering from embarrassment). This does not need to happen as long as communities have the resources to offer various forms of support. For example, a small town newspaper in Michigan's largely rural Upper Peninsula featured an article on a 74-year-old man who has Alzheimer's and is still living in his own home. The front-page article about this man included a picture of him smiling happily as he posed by his garden. He enjoyed a rich social life in large part because of services provided by the Alger County Commission on Aging, including public transportation, aides who come to his home to cook and perform other tasks, and an adult day program that offers a wide range of programs and activities. His daughter gratefully commented, "I don't know what we would do without this. It lets his life be good."

Flourishing communities will be similarly active in seeking ways to continue to engage persons traveling the dementia road in community life. As we show in more detail later, they will establish memory care and creative engagement programs and volunteer within them. They will ensure that the organizations and institutions that form the fabric of the community—religious fellowships, service clubs, sports leagues, and the like—welcome and include persons who have dementia. They will do this in part for altruistic reasons, certainly, but also because they understand that the wider community cannot truly flourish unless its most vulnerable members are also flourishing and that individual lives are diminished when people ostracize (no matter how subtly or indirectly) those who remind them of their own vulnerability.

The Practice of Hospitality

A community comprising persons who understand that each individual is vulnerable and dependent on others—indeed, dependent on relationships with others to be a self—will be defined by the practice of hospitality. Hospitality is commonly reduced to the practice of offering a friendly welcome to friends or strangers who enter a private home, restaurant, hotel, or religious congregation. Here we speak instead of a broader meaning of hospitality, which is centered in the effort to meet the needs of others because we understand that their needs cannot be separated from our own.

A writer once observed that most great stories are variations on one of two themes: a man went on a journey or a stranger came to town. In both versions, hospitality given and received (or perhaps violated) is a central component of the story. The practice of hospitality is "a radical form of reciprocity that creates space for identifying and receiving the stranger as oneself" (Reynolds 2008, 242). In extending genuine hospitality we make ourselves vulnerable, for the one to whom we open ourselves will likely disrupt our routines, make demands on our time, or pull us from our comfort zone. The stranger arrives at our door or enters our life in vulnerability, but once we open the door and allow the stranger to enter, we ourselves become vulnerable.

In the Hebrew Bible, the Israelites are commanded to welcome strangers and sojourners into their household, feeding them and providing for their needs as if they were members of the family (e.g., Lev. 25:23). Christians are likewise exhorted to welcome the stranger, "for by doing so some have entertained angels without knowing it" (Heb. 13:2). Mother Teresa, in opening herself to the poor of Calcutta, saw the presence of Christ in each person she welcomed. And Henri Nouwen once instructed his audience to view every stranger who entered their lives as one specifically sent by God to bring a needed blessing.

In contemporary American society, the practice of hospitality has largely been displaced by the exaggerated value placed on privacy and autonomy. The front porch from which we once exchanged greetings with strolling neighbors and perhaps invited them to stop for a visit has been replaced by the backyard deck or patio, where no one will disturb us. Ask a group of middle-class Americans about the number of people in their lives whom they could comfortably visit without making prior arrangements, and it is likely that few could name more than three or four, most of them relatives. Then ask them about their parents' lives, and many will wistfully recall how unannounced visits were once a part of the fabric of everyday life; now they are fearful of intruding in the lives of even those they regard as close friends. Gated communities stand as stark symbols of our obsession with privacy and security, but the flickering blue light of televisions behind curtained windows and closed doors also speaks of the "electronic moats" that keep the world at bay. Even children have exchanged the spontaneous encounters that school us in the practice of hospitality for the formal structures of play dates and organized sports. We have become distrustful, even fearful, of the stranger, thus weakening the fabric of common community.

Persons who have long placed a premium on preventing other persons, strangers in particular, from disrupting their lives are ill prepared for circumstances in which privacy must be surrendered and autonomy compromised. Older persons moving into frailty or dementia are often loathe to surrender the car keys (a powerful symbol of independence and autonomy) or to consider moving to a retirement community or assisted-living facility, even when the demands of caring for a private home have become exhausting or dangerous. Grief at leaving a beloved home is unavoidable and difficult, of course, but often the resistance stems at least in part from anxiety about sharing social space with other people, especially people different from themselves.

The practice of giving and receiving hospitality—of opening our lives to strangers and those living in circumstances different from our own—is an acknowledgment of our vulnerability and dependence on others. We offer hospitality to the one who needs us because it is the right thing to do and also because it is likely that we will one day be the person requiring someone else's hospitality. We expand our world by welcoming people who are not "just like us," in part because we may face a time when we ourselves are no longer "just like us." In other words, to use Putnam and Feldstein's (2003) language, bonding with others like ourselves is relatively easy; creating bridges between ourselves and those not like us is hard. When we create or sustain relationships with persons who are living with dementia, we may be building bridges to images of our future selves.

Earlier, we offered an image of community as "the place where the person you least want to be with always is." The obligations of community do not require us to be best buddies with that person, but they do require us to interact with him or her with a kind and generous heart. Community teaches us, again and again, that it is not all about us and that, try as we might, we cannot be the authors of our own private universe. We are vulnerable. We are dependent. We can control far less that we wish to believe we can. We must be kind to others and receptive to the stranger because we need such kindness and hospitality from others.

These are not easy practices to learn, particularly within a culture that glorifies autonomy and independence and regards admission of vulnerability as a form of failure. Where can we find a flourishing community centered in friendship, hospitality, and mutual obligation and receive guidance and support for learning these practices? As soon as we begin to think of relationships as defining what it is to be human, we have entered the realm of spirituality, making religious congregations one setting in which we would hope to learn how to be better friends to one another within community.

CHAPTER NINE

Congregations as Schools for Friendship

Most Sundays, a group of very elderly women sits together on a long bench outside their church's library after the worship service. Affectionately called "the Legacy ladies" by many church members because of their residence at a local continuum-of-care retirement community, they wait for the Legacy bus while chatting with one another and with people passing by on the way to the front door. Their church is the last stop for the Sunday morning bus route, so they usually have a lot of time for this kind of casual conversation. They are all mentally sharp, although the years have taken their toll on their bodies, leaving some dependent on walkers or canes; one courageous and determined woman uses both a walker and a portable oxygen tank. In the winter in northeast Wisconsin, temperatures at night can drift down into the "teens below zero," but still these women usually manage to get to church.

One day, a few years ago, they wanted to talk about the sermon, which had focused on kindness in community. "Well," one of them said, "that sermon should be preached at the Legacy!" Others nodded in agreement. We asked them why they thought this. "Because we need to think about kindness."

What they had on their minds was the challenge of dealing with certain residents who were experiencing many of the difficulties of slipping into dementia. The Legacy ladies did not always feel kindly disposed to these fellow residents, and they recognized that they needed to work on this. It was both humbling to witness their honesty in acknowledging the challenge of being kind and inspiring to observe how quickly they grasped that their lives in community demanded their kindness. Having experienced a complex combination of choice and no-choice in giving up independent living in their own homes and turning in their car keys, these women were learning how to live with the kind of close contact with others we associate with college residence halls, the military, hospitals, and residences for the old. However, they had not bargained for the changes that would come in a community of aging people who, like them, had opted to move to the Legacy.[1]

The Legacy ladies were wrestling with some ancient and difficult questions. Why should we care about one another? Why should we value other people, particularly those who seem unable to offer us much in return for our kindness or care? Sociologists speak of social exchange, meaning that people calculate the rewards and costs of relationships, and when the costs exceed the rewards, the relationship ends. Some variations on this formula state that people evaluate their relationship by comparing what each person contributes. If one is contributing more, the relationship is out of balance. Accounting for developmental issues, given that parents generally contribute goods and services to their children long before the children can provide an equitable match, some sociologists calculate return over the long term, observing that "pay off" may come years later, when adult children look after their elderly parents.

Another question bubbling beneath the surface of the Legacy ladies' conversation about kindness in their community concerned their own sense of themselves. They wanted others to know them as what gerontologists sometimes call "high-functioning elders," and they were forthright in admitting concern about identity contamination through their enforced close contact with neighbors who have dementia. This awareness of how the limitations of others threaten our own secure sense of selfhood begins early in life. For example, most adults can vividly recall playground scenes of ostracism of certain children labeled by others as having "cooties" or worse. These are complex challenges and difficult ethical questions, and the Legacy ladies were aware that their faith community was a setting in which they were called to wrestle with them.

Congregations, Demographics, and Priorities

In *Building Healthy Communities through Medical-Religious Partnerships*, Richard Bennett and Daniel Hale (2009) present a case for building collaborations between congregations and health care organizations to strengthen community health education and to advocate for better access to health care for all persons.[2] They note that in the United States, there are more than 330,000 religious congregations. These organizations usually occupy distinctive neighborhood buildings with space, sound equipment, and parking sufficient to support community educational programs. They also have well-established communication systems for getting information to their participants. Many of these institutions already serve their communities in a variety of ways, although, as Bennett and Hale note, the health care industry has been slow to recognize them as partners in community health promotion. Bennett and Hale believe the most important asset that congregations offer to their communities is *human capital*. They write: "This term embraces the rich human resources within most religious institutions. Churches, synagogues, and mosques have established traditions of volunteerism and civic engagement. In every congregation there are members, usually among those who are older, who are willing not only to volunteer their time but also to participate in congregation training programs that enhance their ability to step into leadership roles and to be of service to others in their congregations and communities" (Bennett and Hale 2009, 24).

Even as the U.S. population ages, America's religious communities are aging at a much faster rate. In his study of more than seven hundred congregations representing five Christian denominations (Church of Christ, Southern Baptist, Lutheran, Presbyterian, and Episcopal), Knapp (2003) found that persons age 55 or older made up 20–40 percent of these congregations. In some, the percentage was higher. Most studies that examine religiousness among adults of different ages find that older people "attend church more often than younger people, pray more frequently than younger adults, and read the Bible more often than their younger counterparts" (Krause 2008, 16). This does not, however, mean that people become more religious as they grow older, for cross-sectional studies that compare people by age analyze only age differences, not age changes. Longitudinal studies, which follow the same group of people as they grow older, have produced inconsistent findings. The overall picture seems to be that there are different trajectories through adulthood, with some people declining in religiousness after young adulthood, others remaining the same (whether religious or not), and still others increasing in religiousness but not necessarily in congregational commitments. Of course, the "devil lies in the details" of this research, most notably in the ways it measures religiousness, the representativeness of the people studied, and the range of religious denominations that is included. The last is particularly important in light of Neal Krause's many studies of social relationships in congregations; he has found more people with congregation-based "close companion friends" in conservative compared to liberal religious groups (2008).

What is sometimes referred to as the "graying of the American congregation" reflects many current social trends: more people living longer, the importance of religious faith to today's older adults, and the declining religiosity among younger Americans. A study published in 2010 finds that young adults are presently disaffiliating from religious communities at five to six times the historic rate (Putnam and Campbell 2010). Despite these demographics, however, many congregations still direct a disproportionate percentage of their staffing resources and budgets to the needs of children, youth, and young adults (Knapp 2003; Merchant 2003). Often the argument used for setting such priorities is the need to think of the future. In truth, if current demographic trends continue, the future of many congregations lies with members currently in their fifties, sixties, or seventies.

Although there are still many congregations where older members remain active in leadership positions, there is an unfortunate tendency among some youth-oriented faith communities to take members over the age of 60 for granted or to regard them as if they have graduated from active engagement in congregational life and leadership. One man in his early seventies who had previously held a number of significant offices in his congregation noted that it had been years since he had been asked to hold a leadership position. "I'm not sure I want to do it anymore," he reflected ruefully, "but it would be nice to be asked." If a pastor or church officer is asked why an older member has not been invited to assume a leadership position, a common and sincere answer is, "He's already done so much for the church that he's entitled to a rest" or "She has done more than her fair share; someone else should take a turn." Sometimes, of course, the failure to invite older members to assume leadership positions is classic ageism, expressed in words like: "We need fresh leaders and new ideas if we are going to attract young people."

Likewise, the spiritual needs and challenges of older adulthood too often go unaddressed in sermons and the programmatic life of the faith community. Many members of the clergy appear to believe that younger adults need guidance and instruction in how to apply their faith to the challenges and complexities of everyday life but that older adults have already arrived at such knowledge and understanding. Discussions among pastors suggest that there is a high risk of persons falling away from active engagement with their faith community when they reach the empty-nest years.[3] The most common explanations for this phenomenon are that they believe they have "done their duty" to nurture their children in the faith and no longer feel the need to anchor life in spiritual community or that their weekends are now spent at the cottage, on the golf course, or visiting their adult children. In truth, many likely fall away from active engagement because the faith community is not speaking to their needs and concerns or challenging them to continue in their spiritual growth.

If reaching late midlife can render persons invisible to their faith community, those journeying into old age too often fare even worse, with neglect replaced by condescension. In language that makes us grit our teeth (even though we know it is well-intended), older members are sometimes broken into three categories— "the go-goes," "the slow-goes" and "the no-goes." Gerontologists do in fact apply varying terms to different stages of the journey into old age—*young old, at-risk elders, frail old*—but the language of "the three goes" reinforces stereotypical views of aging as a process of inevitable deterioration and decay. The frail elderly members of the congregation are often described as "our shut-ins," another locution that limits and reduces complex persons to objects of sympathy or even pity. They become the occasional recipients of courtesy visits, leftover altar flowers, and greeting cards made by the children of the congregation. Because they have difficulty participating in congregational life, younger members rarely have the opportunity to know them as individuals with wisdom, wit, and other gifts of friendship to offer. If there is any setting in which the fullness of personhood at each stage of life and in all circumstances should be honored and appreciated, it is within faith communities.

The Practice of Friendship within Congregations: Spiritual Hospitality

Recognizing that personhood is defined by vulnerability and dependence on others, a religious congregation, more than any other community, should understand itself as the setting in which members learn the practice of being friends to one another across the lines of generation and ability. Because they share convictions about values and ultimate meaning in and beyond life, they are not strangers, even if they are not well acquainted in conventional terms. Members are encouraged to view one another as brothers and sisters in faith, carrying the bonds of affection and mutual obligation that define familial relationships. Some religions codify these obligations in specific terms. Judaism, Christianity, and Islam, for example, all dictate the obligation to care for the widows and orphans of the community. More broadly, all major world religions include as a core teaching the ethic of reciprocity (commonly called the Golden Rule) as a moral guide for human relationships, especially relationships within the faith community. We are called to care for others in their need in the same manner we would wish to be cared for if the need were ours.

In *Older Americans, Vital Communities*, Andrew Achenbaum (2005) states that his "bold vision for societal aging" will be realized in part through the actions of aging persons who have experienced spiritual renewal: "Spiritual elders are ideally positioned to play the role of citizen pilgrims in creative ways" (126). Achenbaum imagined these "citizen pilgrims" working to make the world a more hospitable place through a wide variety of civic actions focused on issues ranging from poverty and homelessness, to the environment, health care reform, and peaceful relations among nations. Our focus in this book is more immediate—the care of individuals and families struggling with memory loss—but the impetus for the action is the same.

A primary way in which people care for one another within congregations is by offering their presence in times of need: listening to the person who needs to talk, spending time with the person who is lonely, sitting in companionable silence with someone whose grief they cannot remove or whose pain they cannot take away. Experiences of profound grief or serious illness can isolate a person from the normal routines and web of relationships that define personhood. In spiritual terms, being fully present to someone suffering such circumstances says "God will never leave you alone, and neither will I."

When a member of the faith community travels the dementia road, the gift of our presence is more precious still. Rabbi Dayle Friedman terms this a "ministry of spiritual accompaniment" (2001a). The journey into dementia can be a frightening experience and all too often a lonely one as casual friends visit only on the rare occasions, when they are "in the right mood," or they withdraw completely. The gift of presence to a friend who has dementia in the faith community is a spiritual practice that must be pursued with disciplined intentionality.

Some congregations have organized visitation programs, either in the form of visitation committees whose members make regular calls on shut-ins or one-on-one matches between two members, one of whom is identified as having need of regular visits. In many cases, persons who have dementia are not regarded as candidates for these visitation programs, most likely because those volunteering to serve as visitors do not know how to be present to someone who has dementia and are uncomfortable with the prospect. One woman whose husband has moderately severe Alzheimer's disease noted that no one from the church ever came to visit him until he developed cancer, a "respectable" disease that qualified him for the visitation list.

Anne Basting (2009) challenges the idea that mere "visitation" is the most helpful and appropriate way for a community to be present to a person who has dementia: "*We must remember that memory is social, that the 'self' is relational. To forget this is to ignore one of our best 'cures' for memory loss—creating a net of social memory around a person whose individual control of memory is compromised. This doesn't mean that we should visit people more. This means that people with memory loss need to be reknit into the fabric of our lives. The members of a nursing home staff shouldn't think of a spouse or a son or a daughter or a friend as a visitor. They should think of them as part of their community*" (161).

Being present to a community member in need is a manifestation of hospitality, as is providing practical help and assistance in a time of difficulty. People in the congregation who are ill or injured may need meals prepared, rides to the doctor's office or memory clinic, and other forms of assistance. There may not be family members living nearby to provide such things, or the family may not have sufficient resources to do so. A religious congregation rejects the cultural model that insists that such responsibilities are vested only in family members or personal friends. To share in the life of a congregation is to be present to one another in time of need. In some congregations this kind of practical care for a member in time of need may fall to an organized program, while in others "the ministry of casseroles" may occur through more informal channels.

Illustrating this kind of congregational care, theologian Joel Shuman (2009) described a crisis in the life of his family. Shortly after they had welcomed two toddlers into their home for foster care, his spouse suffered a sudden and serious illness. Members of their congregation, some of whom they did not know personally, stepped in to provide child care, meals, housecleaning, and other essential services. In reflecting on the experience, Shuman wrote: "They were as important to Chris' recovery as the daily antibiotics she was receiving intravenously—literally a healing presence to our household's suffering and disability . . . not only had they taught us what it is to be the church; they had been for us, and continue to be, agents of the wild, faithful God who heals" (38).

After describing the initial feelings of helplessness and panic prompted by his spouse's diagnosis, Shuman said "we called our church." In this he was unusual—for many middle-class persons it is much harder to ask for help than to offer it. Most people have low expectations of their communities, including their faith communities. Paul exhorted Christians to "bear one another's burdens" (Gal. 6:2), but, schooled as many are in the modern virtue of autonomy, "being a burden to others" is framed as a shameful failure. Asking for needed help from others in the community is an acknowledgment of vulnerability, and only this acknowledgment makes genuine community possible.

Such practices of hospitality, of course, should not be limited exclusively to fellow members of the congregation, but it is the setting in which people are most likely to learn such practices. When congregation members offer the gift of their presence or provide practical assistance to a person suffering grief or illness who is not a member of their own family or a close personal friend, they are swimming against the current of the culture of individualism and exposing the myth of personal autonomy. Congregations are rooted in religious beliefs that provide a different story of who and what persons are and how they are to interrelate than the story told by the prevailing culture, and therefore they are settings in which persons can learn the practices of being vulnerable, dependent friends to one another. Stanley Hauerwas and Michael Budde (2000) defined the church as "a school for subversive friendships," and it is exactly these sorts of friendships that must be developed if people are to age together in grace, joy, and hope.

Creative Hospitality: Beyond the Potluck Supper

Faith communities are knit together and strengthened by their traditions, but sometimes these traditions become stultifying, leading to the stereotype that they are set in their ways and unwilling to change. This charge is often unfairly directed at older persons in congregations who are viewed as standing in the way of new ideas and practices. Although there may be a kernel of truth in these stereotypes, in many congregations older adults lead the way in parish renewal and vitalization. As James Ellor notes, "Many older adults are actually experts at handling change" (1995, 277). Nevertheless, it is often easy for groups composed of persons of any age to fall back into old ways of doings things. Scout troops maintain meaningful traditions, but do they still need to sell magazine subscriptions in the twenty-first century? Community service clubs value their weekly lunches, but must they sing the same tired songs every time they gather? Universities have rituals for their students' graduation, but why do they seem incapable of revising the scripts for speeches by chancellors, provosts, and deans? We know an older woman who participates in her congregation's PrimeTimers group, a monthly gathering of older persons (many of whom are in the early stages of memory loss) for a potluck dinner. She questions the need for a potluck every month. In other words, like persons in many community organizations, she wonders why her group cannot be more creative in strengthening its bonds of hospitality and connection with the community.

Some congregations have demonstrated considerable creativity and collaboration in extending hospitality to persons who are living with dementia. The First United Methodist Church of Champaign, Illinois, teamed with Sandy Burgener, professor of nursing at University of Illinois at Urbana-Champaign, to create a multifaceted program for persons with the diagnosis of early-stage dementia. Supported by volunteers from the church, participants (about one-quarter of whom are congregation members) gather for social interaction, cognitive therapy, and practice in traditional Chinese movement, martial arts, and meditation. While the participants engage in these activities, their care partners meet in support groups. The congregation provides some funding to help with "tuition" for those who cannot afford to pay fourteen dollars a day for the program; it has also successfully sought external funding from philanthropic groups. Burgener reports that some people drive an hour each way to participate in the program. She and her colleagues have documented the positive outcomes of participation, in both mental and in physical health and well-being (Burgener et al. 2008).

In Houston, a collaboration of thirteen congregations representing six denominations supports the Amazing Place Memory Care Day Center.[4] People who have mild to moderate memory loss participate in physical exercise, reminiscence, music and art activities, service projects, and much more (Brock 2008). Both Jewish and Christian holidays are celebrated. The center also offers daily Bible study for participants. When the center outgrew its space in a United Methodist Church, a generous donor stepped forward to fund a new building. The new facility includes a chapel.

There are many other possibilities for creative congregational outreach to persons who are living with dementia.[5] Bennett and Hale's (2009) book addressed partnerships between congregations and health care organizations, but such partnerships could also be formed by congregations working with local, county, and state offices on aging, the Alzheimer's Association, adult day programs, and long-term care residences. Given the close ties between many religious organizations and the arts in various forms (McFadden and Ramsey 2010), we can imagine congregations collaborating with local cultural centers to create programs for persons who have dementia and their families, much like the Meet Me at MoMA program at the Museum of Modern Art in New York.[6]

Congregations and religious organizations (e.g., denominational bodies) might also use their camps for respite vacations, designed for persons who have dementia and their care partners. These camps often have well-appointed cabins, dining halls, chapels, and activities areas; many serve families with young children, but could they not also offer a week or two of summer sessions for individuals who have dementia? Trained volunteers and paid staff could craft programs incorporating the arts, music, religious services, and time for enjoyable informal interaction. This might be the type of innovative program that foundations would sponsor, as it could offer new opportunities for friendship, support for care partners, and the blessings of time spent in a beautiful natural environment. Wilz and Fink-Heitz (2008) assessed a program of "assisted vacations" that included caregiving spouses, and they found both immediate and long-term beneficial effects in physical and mental health.

The Congregation as a Center for Ethical Formation

In addition to being a center for the development of practices of spiritual hospitality, a faith community should also be a setting in which members are challenged and guided in matters of ethics and morality. Earlier, we saw how the Legacy ladies struggled with the awareness that they were failing to be friends to their fellow residents who were slipping into dementia. The recently retired person may grapple with the question, "What is my obligation to others now that I am no longer working?" The person who has focused on the accumulation of wealth and material possessions may be asking why these things have not provided greater happiness and comfort, and be ready to engage the question posed by Micah: "What does the Lord require of you but to do justice, and to love kindness, and to walk humbly with your God?" (Mic. 6:8).

Questions of medical ethics and end-of-life care are especially important for members of the congregation journeying into old age. Wider society (the political realm in particular) has not provided a setting in which these ethical questions can be comfortably and safely discussed, and for many people these questions lie close to the heart of their religious convictions. They raise questions about God's intentions for their lives. Are they free to choose to bring their own lives to an end because they no longer find its quality satisfying, as advocates of physician-assisted suicide contend? Or must they seek to stay alive in any and all circumstances, no matter what the financial cost to society, the physical cost to themselves, and the emotional cost to their families, as some insist? When quality of life has diminished because of physical frailty or cognitive decline, are they permitted to opt for "natural death," accepting palliative care but rejecting antibiotics to treat pneumonia? Under what circumstances, if any, do they wish to be treated with "heroic" measures? How does the spiritual principle of good stewardship speak to such decision-making? If a given intervention will extend life only a few months without increasing its quality, and the dollars used to provide such care could be spent on preventive health care for the young, how do the ethical teachings of the faith community guide that decision? Faith communities should be settings in which such questions can be posed, pondered, discussed, and responded to, honestly and openly.

Many religious leaders have been reluctant to encourage such discussions or to offer guidance in these matters. As is true with many other people, speaking directly about decline and death may make them uncomfortable, and speaking about dementia may make them more uncomfortable still. Yet these questions are immediate and urgent for many aging members in congregations. They may have a clear sense of what they wish and do not wish for themselves but be afraid that their children or other family members will oppose these wishes. They may want to express their desires through an advance directive but lack information about how to do so, or they may need to have their wishes blessed by someone who represents spiritual authority to them.

In many decades spent in pastoral ministry, John encountered few people who were deeply fearful of death, but many who were fearful of a "bad" death. Often that fear was expressed through direct and simple words: "If I ever get like that, pull the plug!" But behind those simple words lay strong convictions about God's will and intention for their lives. They understood that life includes suffering and that further suffering likely lay ahead for them. They did not fear pain or death. But they could distinguish between "suffering" and "suffering that serves no greater good," and they wished to be reassured that this distinction was spiritually valid. Sometimes they needed an advocate to assist them in expressing their wishes to children unwilling to give them permission to die. Congregations and those who lead them should facilitate such conversations and offer members ethical guidance in making decisions informed by their beliefs about God's will for their lives.

Spiritual Needs and Opportunities in Later Life

Many younger adults look to their faith communities for practical wisdom and guidance in navigating the multiple demands and challenges of their busy lives—establishing and maintaining relationships, forming values and ethics, childrearing, career development, etc. They view the faith community as a center for family life and are drawn to congregations that offer good-quality programs for their children. This is not to say that they do not also seek connection to the transcendent or guidance in pondering questions of ultimate meaning and purpose, but the practical demands of complex lives tend to push such matters to the periphery.

But in midlife and beyond, with children grown and careers well established or moving toward conclusion, these questions of meaning and purpose become more immediate and open for exploration in new ways. By age 60, most persons are well aware that they have lived more than half of their life expectancy, and mortality is no longer an abstract concept. It is a time when questions about how mortal life relates to the eternal and transcendent become of greater interest.

With many of life's major milestones now in the past, people may come to believe that, as one preacher expressed it, "whatever you were put on earth to do, you likely think that you have pretty much done it by now." But is this necessarily true? With increasing life expectancy, is there the possibility of developing a new sense of passion and purpose in life? The model of retirement that has predominated in our culture for at least fifty years—work hard and earn as much as possible until the age of 65 or 66, then enjoy the reward of a life of leisure—may not be well suited for someone facing another twenty years of relatively good health. With that model being increasingly questioned, some people are pondering existential questions: What will this next stage of life be about? May I put my talents and abilities in the service of others in new ways? Are there talents I have always wished to develop but did not have time to pursue?

The lame joke about the lament of the retiree's spouse—"I married him for better or for worse but not for lunch"—aside, marriages that were largely centered in task sharing, particularly around the needs of children, may need to be renegotiated as couples ponder the prospect of several more decades together and the uncertainties that lie ahead. How do we prepare ourselves to age well? How do we equip ourselves to live as fully and joyously as possible for as long as we can, and how do we prepare ourselves—practically, emotionally, and spiritually—to contend with the possibility of physical or cognitive decline as a part of the journey of aging?

These are but some of the questions asked by those poised at the threshold of early old age. These are the people increasingly being described as being in the third age of life (Weiss and Bass 2002), the time between the first retirement and the onset of frailty. This is a period of life that Marris (2002) described as being "colored by awareness of a powerfully ambiguous future" (39). Memory loss may lurk in that ambiguity; death most definitely will be found there. Sensing this, many people vow to make the most of the gift of energy, health, and time after their first retirement; they want to feel that their lives matter. Some pursue this goal narcissistically, but others seek deeper meaning, through practices that promote spiritual development (Atchley 2009) and through greater service to others.

Congregations must find ways to help their members in the third age to reframe their spiritual journeys in light of the new freedoms they may be experiencing (including the freedom to engage with friendship and service in new ways), their increasing interest in how faith speaks to matters of ultimate concern, and the need to equip themselves for their next stage in life, with both the opportunities and uncertainties it brings. Men and women who have lived outwardly directed lives may seek guidance in exploring the inward dimension through prayer, meditation, or contemplation. Those who are concluding managerial careers may be hungry for hands-on mission and service opportunities. Some who have applied their considerable abilities exclusively to their careers may be delighted by an invitation to place their abilities and experience at the service of the congregation. Others may seek the opportunity to do things far removed from their workplace experience. Some of these people will—perhaps sooner rather than later—receive the diagnosis of mild cognitive impairment or early-stage Alzheimer's disease. This may evoke an acute sense of the need to find ways of defining and meeting their spiritual needs: their need to feel hopeful and validated as persons, to be able to offer love to others, to experience beauty and wonder, and to be assured of God's love (Ryan, Martin, and Beaman 2005).

Those embarking on the journey into life's next stage need both the challenges and the consolations of faith. They should be challenged to reject the prevailing culture's model of the retirement years as a self-indulgent time in which people are relieved of obligations to others in community; instead, they should be inspired to invest themselves in new forms of service. They should be supported in pondering life's meaning and purpose in new ways and in reflecting on what will actually enable them to flourish as they move into their later years. Those who have already learned how to give of themselves to their friends must learn how to accept care and support from their friends in return. And they must be schooled in the comforting, hopeful knowledge that no matter what losses they may face in the coming years, they will remain whole persons and valued members of the community.

Life Review and Spiritual Reminiscence

Growing older leads many people to reflect on their lives—the joys and triumphs, the failures, losses, and disappointments, the milestones along the way. They seek, consciously or not, a coherent narrative of meaning. Most wish to believe that their lives have had purpose and value. Whether framed in humble terms—"I have tried to give a little more than I took"—or in grand descriptions of specific accomplishments that "made a real difference," people seek perspective on the meaning of their lives and how they have mattered to others.

Such reflections need not be an exercise in narcissism if framed in a deeper, spiritual context. In some religious traditions such reflections might be expressed in terms of "how God has worked through my life" or "how God's grace has been present for me." Encouraging and providing a setting for reflecting on one's life journey can be a spiritually enriching activity for older members, allowing them to review their journeys in a manner that brings healing and comfort, as well as hope and direction for the future.

In their guide to facilitating spiritual reminiscence for persons who have dementia, MacKinlay and Trevitt (2006) note that "in many cases, life review gives people an opportunity to reflect on their accomplishments, gives an opportunity to right old wrongs, reconcile with enemies and become ready to die" (24). Since Robert Butler (1963) first gave a positive interpretation to older adults' reminiscence, a process that was once seen as reflecting their obsessive insistence on thinking about the past, gerontologists have embraced the potential for life review as a way of connecting past, present, and future for aging persons (e.g., Gibson 2004). Although others have added the spiritual component to life review (e.g., Morgan 1996), the program developed by MacKinlay and Trevitt lays out a process that provides meaningful spiritual engagement for those whose memories may be compromised but who remain capable of telling stories from their lives that bring joy, reconciliation, comfort, and peace. Their work has shown that older persons who are living with dementia are eager to reflect about meaningful memories but are inhibited because "there is no one to listen" or "my life was ordinary." By providing a setting in which such stories can be shared under the guidance of a skilled and sensitive facilitator, the spiritual community can communicate that each person's story matters because each person matters (Trevitt and MacKinlay 2006).

Honoring through Obligation

Religions vary in the spiritual obligations that adherents are commanded to honor. For Muslims, the Five Pillars of Islam constitute such an obligation. Jews are *metzuveh* (commanded) to honor the sacred covenant and the commandments, both ritual and ethical. Roman Catholic Christians are obligated to participate in the Mass on Sunday and on Holy Days of Obligation. Protestant Christianity is less centered in formal obligations beyond, as one theologian dryly expressed it, "sincerely trying to be nice," although this varies among Protestant traditions.

Friedman (2008) argues for the importance of holding elders entering into dementia accountable to the obligations of their faith. As in other religions centered in specific obligations, Judaism offers what Friedman terms "sliding-scale" obligation to those whose physical or cognitive limitations preclude complete observance:

> A person who is old or weak and unable to stand may recite the *Amidah* (standing) prayer sitting down or even prone. . . . An individual who cannot speak may discharge the obligation by mentally reciting the prayers or by meditating upon them.

A person who does not have the endurance to complete the entire liturgy may abbreviate the Amidah.

What is most significant about this "sliding scale" model of obligation for elders is that, once obligated, we remain so, even in the face of diminished capacity. All of the social and personal benefits of being *metzuveh* continue to accrue, because as long as we perform the mitzvah to the extent of our ability, we are considered to have fully discharged the responsibility. (19)

Friedman notes that Rabbi Abraham Joshua Heschel taught that it is through the experience of being obligated that we truly exist. How tragic, then, that so often persons who are aging or journeying into dementia are relieved of all obligations by well-intentioned persons, including their religious leaders. Essentially they are told, no matter how kindly, that their existence no longer matters to God or to other people.

To the contrary, we honor the personhood of our friends who have dementia by continuing to have expectations of them and by adjusting their obligations as necessary rather than stripping them of all obligations. If community, including spiritual community, is a web of relationships among vulnerable, dependent persons, then all who participate in community have obligations to one another.

Creative congregations that are intent on honoring their older members will work to identify the ways in which these cherished members can still contribute. Those with limited mobility can assist with "telephone trees" and prayer chains or can mentor younger members. People who have dementia, even significant cognitive loss, are often able to say the words to familiar prayers and sing beloved hymns, contributing to corporate worship. Many congregations have developed accommodations that enable full inclusion of members with impaired sight or hearing; it is equally possible to accommodate persons with memory impairment. In one setting, a person who had significant memory impairment was able to read the scripture lesson aloud to the worshiping congregation while an assistant moved his finger along the lines of the text so that the reader would not lose her place. A local pastor described a dedicated member whose cognitive abilities have declined: "Physically she's just fine. She's our chair of stewardship. It is an act of loving mercy that she is still in that position. We all know what's going on, and we work around it. She loves doing this and she's a faithful giver to the church; I just couldn't tell her she had to resign. The down side is that the committee hasn't worked to its fullest potential. We can handle that in the short term, though. She has only a year left of her six-year term as chair."

In a growing literature on voluntarism among older adults, researchers note that serving others gives people a sense of purpose and connects them to people in a meaningful way (Okun and Shultz 2003; Shmotkin, Blumstein, and Modan 2003). In fact, several studies have shown that older people volunteer because of the opportunities to form friendships (e.g., Rook and Sorkin 2003). Persons who are living with dementia should also have the opportunity to meet their religious obligations and to reap the rewards of meaning and purpose that helping others can offer. In addition, they should not be excluded from the health benefits of voluntarism now widely documented by researchers (e.g., Brown et al. 2003; Morrow-Howell et al. 2003; Oman, Thoresen, and McMahon 1999).

Finally, just because a person's dementia has progressed to the point that he or she needs residential care does not mean that the opportunity to be of service to others or to meet one's faith tradition obligations must end. For example, Rabbi Dayle Friedman described how she helped frail nursing home residents "adopt" a young Ethiopian Jew who had fled his country to Israel. Volunteers (often friends from the community) helped them write letters and raise money for this young man. They also prayed regularly for him. Friedman wrote that "the nursing home residents had transcended their roles as recipients of care. They had become *redeemers*" (2001b, 297).

A Community of Blessing

If a congregation—regardless of its particular religious tradition—is understood as a web of spiritual relationships among vulnerable, dependent persons, then it must also serve as a "community of blessing." In its life together, the congregation blesses newborn babies through ritual or sacrament. It offers blessings to those who marry or enter partnership together. It grieves those who pass to death and offers blessings as that cherished person enters the realm of unknown mystery. Community participants bless one another through their presence and mutual care. Ideally, they offer blessings to one another across the lines of gender, race, political affiliation, sexual orientation, age, and ability. They bless one another because they are friends who value one another, friends who hold a story in common, and friends who share important beliefs, values, and convictions. Blessed by one another's friendships, they are strengthened to reach out in friendship to offer their blessings to those outside of the congregation. Congregations are called to be schools for subversive friendship, subversive because they do not follow the script of the prevailing culture, which argues that there should always be a practical return for friendship.

Spiritual communities confer blessings across the lines of generation in both directions. The old offer blessings to the young, even though they may not fully approve of or understand youthful attitudes or lifestyles. The young bless the old with their very presence, no matter how dimly they comprehend the experience of being elderly.

> On the very cold first Sunday in January, the Legacy ladies were lined up on their bench as usual. An adorable little girl was leaving church with her mother. The girl, about age 8, was dressed in a way that would not have looked out of place in the nineteenth century, with her little wool coat and hat. She went up to each of the Legacy ladies, solemnly extended her hand to theirs, and worked her way down the line, saying "Happy New Year," "Happy New Year," "Happy New Year." Of course, they were delighted to receive her blessing, and of course they replied "and Happy New Year to you, too." After she had greeted them all, she ran back to her mother saying, "Can I say Happy New Year to other people?" "Yes," her mother said. And so, we received—and gave—our blessing, too. We received it from the little girl and from watching her with the Legacy ladies. It was a blessing that went beyond wishing us a happy new year, for it evoked a profound sense of gratitude for being a part of a community in which a little girl could so freely approach a gathering of old ladies to wish them a happy new year and, in turn, invite them to give their blessings to her.

Participants in congregations are friends to one another because they understand that they are vulnerable and therefore in need of friends. They are friends to one another because they hold the conviction—the faith—that being friends to one another is, in the end, the purpose of their lives.

Faith is something we experience not only cognitively but also physically and emotionally. Faith is not something that can ever be fully comprehended or mastered, only lived gratefully and joyfully in communion with others. Faith, in the end, is not about what is lost with the passing of the years (although those losses are real); it is about placing those losses in the perspective of those things than nothing can take away or diminish. Paul wrote, "For I am convinced that neither death, nor life, nor angels, nor rulers, nor things present, nor things to come, nor powers, nor height, nor depth, nor anything else in all creation will be able to separate us from the love of God" (Rom. 8:38–39). We can add dementia to Paul's list: it cannot rob life of meaning, value, joy, or friendship, and it should not be permitted to rob someone of obligations to others or of his or her role as a valued, contributing member of the faith community.

CHAPTER TEN

The Things That Abide

When I lately stood with a friend before [the cathedral of] Amiens,
and he beheld with awe and pity that monument of giant strength
in towering stone, and of dwarfish patience in minute sculpture,
he asked me how it happens that we can no longer build such
piles? I replied: "Dear Alphonse, men in those days had convictions, we moderns have opinions, and it requires something more
than an opinion to build a Gothic cathedral."

Heinrich Heine, *The Salon*

Duke Divinity School professor Stanley Hauerwas argues that it is possible to
assess where a society invests its faith by observing which buildings are most
imposing and impressive.[1] For most of human history, places of worship—the
Great Temple of Jerusalem, Saint Peter's Basilica, the Masjid al Haram Mosque
in Mecca, the Salt Lake City Tabernacle—dominated city skylines and symbol-
ized humanity's deepest convictions and highest hopes. In postwar America,
a new kind of cathedral began to appear on the landscape—huge, monolithic
buildings housing corporate offices and research facilities, representing the
faith we invested in technological and economic progress to lead us to the promised land of prosperity. In our own era, Hauerwas suggests, the most impressive
"cathedrals" are the sprawling medical centers. The Mayo Clinic has become the
new Lourdes, where we invest our faith and our hope of being delivered from
suffering and death.

Whether or not they understand themselves to be religious, those who journey with a cherished friend or family member who has dementia will have am-
ple reason to ponder life's deepest themes and questions. How do we place the
present experience of that friend in the broader context of a life imbued with
meaning and value? What are the deeper resources that can sustain the friend—
and us—in times of challenge or the painful reality of suffering? What endures
beyond the transience of mortal life? Paul (1 Cor. 13:13) famously spoke of the
three things that abide—faith, hope, and love. We consider each of these in turn.

What Is Faith?

Paul Tillich (1957) insisted that "there is hardly a word in the religious language, both theological and popular, which is subject to more misunderstandings, distortions and questionable definitions than the word 'faith.'" He then offered his own definition of faith as "the state of being ultimately concerned" (1). Tillich was seeking a definition that could lay fair claim to being universal, embracing both those who consider themselves religious and those who do not. All persons have something that they look to for ultimate meaning and purpose in life. It may be the nation-state, the family, or the tribal group. It may be personal power, prestige, or material success. It may be a code of ethics. Or it may be a higher power acknowledged to be God. Whoever or whatever people look to for ultimate meaning is the object of their faith.

As Tillich wryly observed, religious groups in particular offer a wide array of definitions of what it means to have or to hold a faith, often associating it with subscribing to a set of beliefs or doctrines—to "have faith" is to believe particular things about God or to believe them in a particular way. Here we speak of faith more broadly, as a relationship with an external source of meaning—an ultimate concern—that commands commitment, loyalty, fidelity, and trust. To be faithful to a spouse, partner, or friend is not merely to believe in that person's existence. To have faith, whether in a supreme deity or in a friend, is to invest trust, loyalty, and commitment in that ongoing relationship.

In an earlier chapter we discussed Martin Buber's distinction between I-Thou and I-it relationships. I-Thou describes relationships with other beings (whether persons or God) who are complete in themselves, neither reducible nor fully knowable. These are relationships we are not free to manipulate or control. I-it describes relationships with material objects that can be understood and reduced to component parts—items we are free to use to our purposes and pleasures. Objects of faith can be roughly separated into the same two categories. It is certainly possible to invest a kind of faith in an "it." We speak, for example, of having faith that our car will get us home through bad weather or faith that medical technology will cure us of a disease. Here faith is associated with trust in human ability to design and manufacture devices that will reliably fulfill their intended function.

University of Montana philosopher Albert Borgmann (1984) draws the distinction between such devices and what he terms "focal things." We live in a world of technological devices that meet our needs and serve our desires without demanding anything from us in return or even requiring that we understand them. We press the "play" button on a CD player and music comes forth. We turn on the computer and a world of information appears before our eyes. A tray slides our body into a magnetic-resonance-imaging device at the hospital and the internal structure of our body is revealed. We click the thermostat on the wall and the central-heating system brings our home to the desired temperature. Most of us have no knowledge of how these devices work, but we trust them—we invest a kind of faith in them—to perform their appointed function to our benefit.

Borgmann contrasts such devices with focal things, which require us to develop a set of skills in order to enjoy their benefits. A wood stove, for example, is a focal thing because it makes relational demands of us that a central-heating system does not. We must secure, split, and stack the firewood. We must learn how to start and tend the fire. Vigilance is required to make certain that the fire does not die out or escape the stove. The pattern of our day must be adjusted so that we are present to add more wood when it is needed. Unlike a device, a focal thing demands that the user establish an ongoing relationship with it. In this sense it can mirror the faith we invest in another person or in God because it requires us to adopt ongoing relational practices that help form our identity as a self.

Because such focal practices become so interwoven with selfhood over time, persons living with advanced dementia often retain their ability to practice them even when cognitive faculties are greatly diminished. Because they are relational, these deeply practiced acts remain intact long after other abilities have been lost. We could cite numerous examples of persons no longer able to live independently who remain able to play the piano or violin, entering a blissful state that resembles transcendent worship. Practicing their continuing relationship with a focal thing moves them both deep within themselves and beyond themselves at the same time.

Faith is concerned with the things that abide, the things that cannot be taken from us by immediate circumstances, because their essence lies not in what we intrinsically possess but in who and what we are in relationship to the object of our faith. As dementia progresses, a person may ultimately forget how to play even a cherished musical piece with which he or she has shared a deep relationship for decades. Similarly, within advanced dementia a person may one day forget the identity of a beloved friend, and even the most devout person may forget God. But the friend—and God—will not forget the person, so the relationship continues, and the selfhood formed by that relationship also abides.[2]

Faith, the I-Thou relationship in which we invest our trust, loyalty, and commitment, connects us with those things beyond us that are greater than ourselves—the divine, the holy, the created order, art and beauty, the family of humankind, the ethical ideal of the good—and sets our personal experiences in a broader and deeper context. In particular, faith provides a context that helps us to cope with loss, pain, suffering, and grief. If a person has invested trust only in his or her own abilities, material achievements, or social status rather than in external relationships, then everything that provides life with meaning and value is threatened by serious illness, dementia in particular. As Jesus counseled, "Do not store up for yourselves treasure on earth, where moth and rust consume and thieves break in to steal; but store up for yourselves treasure in heaven, where neither moth nor rust consumes and where thieves do not break in and steal. For where your treasure is, there your heart will be also" (Matt. 6:19–21). Living by faith, whether or not that faith is specifically religious, means investing ultimate concern, and the meaning that accompanies it, in relationships rather than possessions.

Faith is expressed less through formal beliefs than through disciplined practices that demonstrate loyalty and reinforce commitment to the object of that faith. Faith in a spouse or partner, for example, is demonstrated in the effort to "love, honor, and obey"; to seek the partner's good to the same degree that we seek our own. For Jews, faith is expressed through the ongoing effort to honor and live by the *mitzvot*, following "the ritual and ethical commandments given in the Torah and applied by Jews through the generations" (Friedman 2001b, 291). For Christians, faith is the ongoing effort to follow the command of Jesus to "follow me" in the way of self-giving love. For Muslims faith is expressed through the disciplined practice of the Five Pillars of Islam. Faith is not merely a conviction held, but a life lived.

Some will quickly protest that religious faith cannot be reduced to practices alone, which is a fair objection. Each world religion offers a unique narrative that frames life's meaning, value, and purpose through sacred stories that are transmitted from generation to generation, and each offers core beliefs and convictions to which adherents are called to subscribe. But the narrative of sacred story and the beliefs and convictions which accompany that narrative in themselves provide a relational context that forms and shapes selfhood over time.

Through the sacred stories of a faith tradition, people are able to set their own experiences—including experiences of doubt, anxiety, and suffering—within the context of a narrative that began long before they were born and that will continue beyond their death. They read the stories of others in their faith tradition who suffered similar travails but found comfort, healing, and hope in God or other members of the faith community. They hear the accounts of those who underwent great suffering but who, through their faith, found meaning in that suffering that provided the strength and courage to endure. Stories of their individual lives become part of a much larger story, one that enables people to make sense of suffering by setting it in the context of ultimate meaning, in which life triumphs over death, hope over despair, and good over evil.

In most religions, the primary practice that shapes and forms selfhood is corporate worship. In worship, people hear the sacred stories of the faith tradition. Worship invites participants to affirm their convictions about what gives human life meaning, purpose, and dignity. In this congregate setting, people can experience themselves not solely as isolated individuals but as members of a community not bound by geography or time. Worshippers encounter a spiritual center that can anchor and guide their lives by telling the story of what gives purpose and meaning to mortal life.

The specific relational practices of worship vary tremendously among faith communities, but, like the relationship formed with a "focal thing," they constitute a process of spiritual formation that over time becomes deeply integrated into selfhood in a manner that can endure through the losses that accompany aging, including cognitive losses. Anyone who has observed or participated in a worship service in a skilled-care facility has witnessed how these practices can abide, even for persons who have advanced dementia. The person who is no longer able to speak in complete sentences may be able to recite a sacred text—Psalm 23, for example—in its entirety or sing the verses of a beloved hymn. Once, during a Roman Catholic Mass, when the Host was distributed during the Eucharist, we watched in wonder as a man who was generally unresponsive lifted up his head and opened his mouth like, as a family member expressed it, "a young bird in the nest about to be fed." According to the tenets of the faith he had lived for so many years, he was intimately connected to the transcendent in that moment.

Rabbi Dayle Friedman, who served for twelve years as director of chaplaincy services at the Philadelphia Geriatric Center, describes religious ritual as an "orienting anchor in the midst of confusing, alienating losses, changes, and stresses" (2003, 135). It affirms meaning for participants, and it "pierces isolation and creates community" (136). Regular religious ritual in residential care homes "can infuse time with significance" (137), for these are places where time often weighs heavily on people. "Is it Shabbes?" people ask. "Is it time for church?" In most religious congregations, not only does the worship service offer an anchor in time, but the informal interactions before and after the service have a similar function. Friends chat, drink a cup of coffee, and feel like they are a part of a larger community. Therefore, just as most congregations have some kind of fellowship time following services, progressive dementia-care residences include this time for informal interaction in conjunction with religious worship.[3] Both the formal religious rituals that connect worshippers to one another and to the faithful through the ages, as well as informal practices like coffee and cookies after a religious service, are meaningful and need not be denied to persons who are living with dementia.

Michael DeLashmutt (2009) compares the knowledge of God to knowledge of a piece of music because it is a knowledge that grows out of participation. He contrasts this with knowledge that comes from sensing one's physical state (e.g., hunger), relational knowledge (between persons), and objective knowledge (the stapler on my desk is black). Using the music analogy, he writes:

> Knowing a piece of music, as a musician, involves a kind of participation within the music. Yet as anyone who has ever played an instrument can attest to, it is often a kind of knowledge which is exceedingly difficult to pin down. When I used to play the piano, I would at times lose myself in playing a well-rehearsed song. Yet as soon as I would reflect upon the task of playing the piece, I would often cease being able to play the very same music that only seconds before had felt second-nature. Like the knowledge of music, the knowledge of God is a kind of knowledge which can never be fully attained. It is a knowledge that always leads to a kind of unknowing. (591)

We would add that even as such knowledge of God can never be fully attained, neither can it easily be erased by cognitive decline. The formal and informal practices of faith provide continuity of the self because they are deeply rooted in relationships—both with other persons and with the transcendent—that no loss can completely strip away. They constitute the "treasure in heaven" of which Jesus spoke.

The Book of Job is generally interpreted as a reflection on suffering, innocent suffering in particular. But it also provides guidance—primarily through negative example—of how to be present as a faithful friend to one who suffers. After Job suffers a sequence of disastrous losses and afflictions, Job's three friends seek, through lengthy discourses, to justify God to Job. They attempt to provide an explanation that will somehow make sense of senseless tragedy.

In her commentary on Job, Carol Newsome (1996) notes:

Perhaps the most prominent issue in the dialogues is that of the proper conduct of a person in suffering. For the friends, suffering is an occasion for moral and religious self-examination and reflection. Although there is no single "meaning" for suffering, it is to be understood in some way as a communication from God. For the wicked, it is judgment (15:20–43); for the ethically unsteady, it is a warning (33:14–30); for the morally immature, it is a form of educational discipline (5:17–19); and for the righteous, it is simply something to be borne with the confidence that God will eventually restore well-being (4:4–7). . . . Implicit in the friends' view is the assumption that God is always right and that it is the human being who must make use of the experience to learn what God is trying to communicate. (334)

It is not our purpose to explore the complex theological questions raised by suffering but rather to note that even as Job's friends retreated to the conventional piety of their day to "explain" why Job suffered, it is not uncommon in our own time for well-intentioned friends to offer sentimental clichés ("everything happens for a reason" or "God never gives us more than we can handle") to someone who suffers misfortune or loss through no discernable fault of his or her own. Job's friends fail to enact the essential role of a friend, which is simply to be present to him in his suffering and, through the gift of their caring presence, help make the burden bearable.

If a friend is diagnosed with early-stage Alzheimer's disease or some other form of dementia, it is an understandable impulse to wish to "fix" the situation by offering words of justification ("I know that God has some higher purpose for this"), denial ("Maybe the doctor is wrong; you seem fine to me!"), or empty hopes ("You are going to be one of the lucky ones for whom it never gets worse!") It is far more helpful, and faithful, to offer the simple gift of our presence than hollow words born of our own fears. The message that needs to be heard is, "You will not have to walk this road alone; I am here for you and will always be here for you." A person of religious faith can offer his or her friend the comforting conviction that "neither death, nor life, nor angels, nor rulers, nor things present, nor things to come, nor powers, nor height, nor depth, nor anything else in all creation will be able to separate us from the love of God" (Rom. 8:38–39). Our faithful presence bears witness to this conviction. The greatest gift of faith to share with a friend who suffers is the conviction that the friendship will endure and that the friend will be cherished regardless of the form the suffering may take.

Hope and Optimism

The words *hope* and *optimism* are often used interchangeably (even in some dictionaries), when in fact they describe different phenomena. To be optimistic is to expect a positive outcome based on observable facts or previous experience. If an economist claims, "I am optimistic that the financial markets will recover by the spring," he is speaking out of his experience with previous market cycles and his analysis of current economic indicators. If a surgeon assures her patient that she is optimistic about the outcome of a surgical procedure, her optimism is based on having performed many similar operations that had positive outcomes. That we sometimes use the phrase "unwarranted optimism" in itself suggests that optimism is normally based on demonstrable evidence.

The diagnosis of Alzheimer's disease appears to provide little ground for optimism. It is a progressive disease; it will get worse. Medications and other interventions may slow the rate of the disease's progress, but they cannot cure it. It is a terminal illness; it will ultimately lead to death. The person receiving the diagnosis of AD confronts the certainty that he or she faces a frightening course of cognitive decline, which will bring profound suffering and loss. To say to such a person "I know that everything is going to be just fine" is dishonest. Everything is not going to be just fine.

Are there any grounds for optimism within the diagnosis of Alzheimer's? Certainly there are, if we expand our definition of optimism. Optimism, for example, can be expressed that the person will experience a full and flourishing life within the reality of cognitive loss. One can be optimistic that life will continue to offer laughter, pleasure, joy, and love. Above all, there can be optimism that those who travel the dementia road will continue to be valued members of their communities and that their friendships will continue, so they will not travel this road alone. But note that none of these sources of optimism stems from the person's own resources or a confident expectation that medical science will cure the disease. This form of confidence is based on continuing relationships of loyalty, commitment, and trust and should therefore properly be termed *hope* rather than *optimism*.

Hope grows from "the conviction of things not seen" (Heb. 11:1). Whereas optimism is based on trust in one's own agency ("I know that if I study hard I can pass this test") or observable phenomena, hope grows from faith in our relationship with other persons or in a transcendent agent that will prevail even in the face of human weakness or failure. For a biologist, this may take the form of faith in the force of life itself to survive and flourish despite the environmental damage caused by humans. A person who rejects the formal constructs of religion may yet affirm a "loving intent" to the cosmos. When the odds of prevailing against an enemy whose force appears too overwhelming to permit optimism (one might think of England in the darkest days of World War II), hope may spring from faith in the human spirit or national character. We are optimistic when what we can observe points toward achievement of the desired outcome. We dare to hope when all that we can observe points toward failure or defeat.

For the religious person, the ultimate source of all hope is God. The sacred stories of many faith traditions include accounts of a God who acts to heal the sick, liberate the enslaved, overturn the reign of dictators, and bring justice to the poor and oppressed in circumstances in which human agency alone could not achieve these ends. "I am the Lord, and I will free you from the burdens of the Egyptians and deliver you from slavery to them. I will redeem you with an outstretched arm and with mighty acts of judgment" (Exod. 6:6). Religious hope grows from the conviction that God can do what human beings cannot and that God's perfect love remains with us no matter what challenges or losses we may face.

Although hope is not always rooted in religious faith, it necessarily brings us into the realm of the spiritual. Scholars in recent years have expended much energy attempting to differentiate spirituality from religion and to define both clearly enough so as to defend their differentiation.[4] It is not our purpose here to wade into that complex territory. For now, we return to the work of MacKinlay (2001), who defines relational spirituality as "that which lies at the core of each person's being, an essential dimension which brings meaning to life. [It is] constituted not only by religious practices, but understood more broadly, as relationship with God, however God or ultimate meaning is perceived by the person, and in relationship with other people" (52). MacKinlay and Trevitt (2006) describe spirituality as ultimate meaning mediated through religion, the arts, the environment, and relationships of intimacy. The self is in continuous relationship with sources of meaning, beauty, and joy. Whatever language or images are employed, to understand one's nature as spiritual is to experience one's individual life as part of a greater, benevolent pattern of life in which we participate and are valued.

We may hope that others will be there for us when we need them, which is an expression of faith in our friends. We may hope that we will be granted the gift of divine comfort and assurance, which is an expression of faith in God. More broadly, we dare to hope that even if life is marked by decline, loss, and suffering, we will continue to participate in the greater life of the transcendent realm. We may call it heaven, eternal life, the mind of God, or the heart of the cosmos, but living in hope expresses the conviction that we participate in it and will continue to do so even beyond mortal death. Hope is rooted in the conviction that whatever might befall us, "All shall be well and all shall be well and all manner of thing shall be well" (Julian of Norwich, quoted in Beer 1998).

The fear and anxiety about dementia that we described in Chapters 6 and 7—fear and anxiety for the self and for the other—can undermine hope, even as they can also undermine the faith that gives rise to hope. When one we cherish begins the journey into dementia, hope may be overcome by fear and anxiety. A friend can offer the gift of faith to replenish the hope that has been crushed. By demonstrating continuing loyalty and commitment to the relationship, a friend offers reassurance that the one beginning this frightening new journey will not travel it alone because the person's spiritual core remains a part of the web of relationship, both human and divine, that is the source of faith and hope. By offering loving presence, people can help their frightened friends to experience how "love casts out fear" (1 John 4:18).

Learning the Ways of Love

One of us had the privilege of hearing a lecture by the late Henri Nouwen (1932–96), who was then living at Daybreak, a L'Arche community in Canada. Nouwen, a Catholic priest, left an active, successful academic life teaching in settings like Harvard and Yale, to live in a L'Arche community and minister to mentally handicapped people. Founded by Jean Vanier in France, "L'Arche communities, family-like homes where people with and without disabilities share their lives together, give witness to the reality that persons with disabilities possess inherent qualities of welcome, wonderment, spirituality, and friendship. Perhaps an extraordinary notion in our fast-paced and consumer-driven society, L'Arche believes that these qualities, expressed through vulnerability and simplicity, actually make those with a disability our real teachers about what is most important in life: to love and to be loved."[5]

In his lecture, Nouwen told the story of how he was instructed to cancel a demanding international speaking schedule in order to provide daily care for one of the most severely disabled members of the community. He described his initial resentment at this assignment, which prevented him from continuing what he regarded as his important work. But over time he came to see the man for whom he cared as the most important spiritual teacher of his life. Even though Adam could not speak, Nouwen learned to read the language of his eyes, and he saw in those eyes perfect love for him. An acclaimed spiritual teacher, Nouwen had never known such an experience of being completely and perfectly loved, and it gave him a new understanding of what it means to be perfectly loved by God.[6]

As Nouwen's love for Adam grew, Adam taught him a second important lesson about love. There was no way in which Adam could "earn" love from Nouwen or anyone else. Adam could not speak or feed himself; even the most basic functions of self-care were beyond his ability. The only reason to love Adam was for his very existence as a precious child of God—in the term Nouwen preferred, he saw in Adam "the Beloved." Adam taught Nouwen that love does not need to be earned and indeed cannot be earned; none of us can claim to be "worthy" of love from God or from another person. It is a gift that we can but accept humbly and gratefully.

Adam helped Nouwen to realize that despite his widespread reputation as a spiritual teacher of great wisdom, a part of him was still driven to seek not just recognition, but love, through his acclaimed books and lectures. Adam taught him how to focus less on doing and more on simply being, to slow life's pace and concentrate on the joy of being able to love and the gift of being loved in return.

In our culture, the word *love* is used in a bewildering assortment of ways, most commonly associated with an emotion related to passion, affection, and attachment. We speak of "falling in (or out of) love" or of being "lovesick." We name as objects of our love not only our chosen partner, but also chocolate, Shakespeare, and the Green Bay Packers. Here we speak of love as active concern for the well-being of another that makes us willing to give of ourselves without counting the cost. Or, in the words of de Rivera, love is "the underlying motivational concern for the other" (1989, 402). In Chapter 7, we discussed de Rivera's concept of the "third self," the state in which we set aside the always-present fear for the self to fully love another. But how do we do this?

Miroslav Volf, Henry B. Wright Professor at Yale University Divinity School and director of the Yale Center for Faith and Culture, has written extensively on forgiveness and reconciliation. A Croatian by birth, Volf is well acquainted with the unspeakable atrocities human beings perpetrate on one another and the difficulty of granting forgiveness to those who have so grievously wronged us. His characterization (1996) of reconciliation as a "drama of embrace" is equally descriptive of the manner in which any person who is fearful for the self may reach out to another in love. An embrace, whether physical or metaphorical, has four component parts: opening the arms, waiting, closing the arms, and opening them again.

The first "act"—*opening the arms*—creates space in one's life for the other, indicating "I do not want to be myself only; I want the other to be part of who I am and I want to be part of the other" (141). Volf notes that the self that is "full of itself" cannot move toward or receive the other—opening the arms requires pushing back the self in order to issue an invitation for the other to enter. The inviting self does not demand that the other enter the space created. Rather, it issues what Volf calls a "soft knock" on the other's door.

The second act in the drama of embrace is *waiting*. Without the waiting, an embrace may be perceived as an act of violence, actively forcing one's self on the other. "If embrace takes place, it will always be because the other has desired the self just as the self has desired the other" (143). One waits because, while the embrace may have originated in the self, it cannot be fulfilled unless the other offers relational reciprocity.

In act 3 the drama is fulfilled in *closing the arms*. Now the two persons—the one who initiated and the other who accepted the invitation—are in mutually chosen reciprocal relationship. Each is embracing and each is being embraced. They may not be giving and receiving equally, but each is giving and receiving, and each has entered the space of the other. Volk emphasizes the importance of maintaining a "soft touch," in which the initiator does not seek to crush or assimilate the other. "In an embrace the identity of the self is both preserved and transformed, and the alterity [otherness] of the other is both affirmed as alterity and partly received into the ever changing identity of the self" (143).

The final act of the drama is *opening* the arms again. The goal is not for individual identities to be lost or swallowed up, but for each to return to its own identity enriched by the presence of the other and carrying the knowledge that the relationship continues even when they are apart.

Having described the structure of the embrace, Volk goes on to examine notable features of a "successful" embrace, including the manner in which it affirms the fluidity of our identities. Each self is in a continuous process of dynamic change as we act and are acted on by others in community. "Our selves and our communities are like our domiciles in which we feel at home, and yet keep remodeling and rearranging, taking old things out and bringing new things in. . . . Things we encounter 'outside' become a part of the 'inside'" (145). No encounter leaves us unchanged; it is through relationships that the self is formed and reformed. He notes also the risk of embrace: "I open my arms, make a movement of the self toward the other . . . and do not know whether I will be misunderstood . . . or whether my action will be appreciated, supported and reciprocated" (147).

In seeking to actively love a friend who has dementia, Volf's "drama of embrace" can be helpful as both physical description and metaphor. Physical touch is often a greatly appreciated expression of loving relationship for a person who is living with dementia. But if one is to honor that person's selfhood, the right to embrace should not be assumed. Perhaps this is a day in which physical touch is threatening, even frightening or painful. Love may be better expressed through the soft knock of invitation, opening one's arms and waiting for the friend to respond. Likewise in conversation it is wise, and loving, to begin with gentleness and to seek permission rather than assume it. "Hello! It is good to see you! Is this a good time to visit? May I come in?"

It is also good to be mindful of Volf's insistence that an embrace is always mutual. Each party enters the space of the other, and each is open to being enriched and changed by the encounter. Even as a one-way embrace may be experienced as invasive, violent, or controlling, affection given without the joyous hope of receiving love in return becomes a mere duty or act of charity rather a genuine offering of love. We have noted before that many persons who are living with dementia possess an extraordinary sensitivity to the emotions of others—what is sometimes crudely termed a "B.S. detector." Glad-handing and bear-hugging are empty and hollow gestures when they are devoid of a genuine love that is mindful of the sacred, irreducible mystery of the other and is genuinely open to receiving blessings from the encounter.

Love, Paul wrote, "bears all things, believes all things, hopes all things, endures all things" (1 Cor. 13:7). Love is commitment for the long haul; it does not permit the possibility of abandonment. Love gives of itself, expecting nothing in return, but remains ever open to the surprising, unexpected gifts that may be received. Love chooses to give of itself in relationships with others because that is what love cannot help but do. To love someone who is traveling into dementia is to be granted the gift of learning wonderful new things about both giving and receiving love. By sharing one's faith with such a friend, one's faith can be deepened. To share one's hope with such a friend is to have one's own hope renewed. And to share one's love with such a friend is to discover new dimensions of what love is, and what love can be.

More than a year after Annie's death from AD, her husband, daughter, son, and granddaughter attended a conference about care for persons who are living with dementia. They were there in part to express their gratitude to those who had cared for Annie, and for them, during her final months of life in a skilled-care facility. But they were also there to offer their testimony of how love can blossom in new ways within the journey of dementia.

They had always been a close and devout family, and they were devastated by Annie's rapid decline. Annie had been in every sense the family matriarch—a wealthy woman of indomitable will. Like many women in her cohort, Annie had been taught that it was unseemly to display her emotions, which sometimes led others to see her as cold or distant. But within the journey of dementia, dimensions of Annie that had been carefully controlled all of her life began to emerge. She became openly affectionate, spontaneous, and playful. These changes were initially disconcerting to her family, an indication that "mom was no longer herself." But bit by bit they learned to give and receive love in ways that Annie's previous restraint had not permitted, exchanging hugs and kisses freely, with her and with one another. While there was grief over the loss of her cognitive abilities, there was also joy in the new freedom that had been granted to her and to them. They prayed together, played together, laughed together.

When Annie was first admitted to the dementia unit of the skilled-care facility, fear all but eclipsed her family's ability to love her. Over time they learned that her dementia was not something to fear, but rather a new experience within their loving journey together. The "drama of embrace" they experienced through Annie's final months proved a blessing to her and to them. They attended the conference because they wanted to tell their story to families just beginning this journey. They wanted them to know that they should be ruled not by fear, but by love.

CHAPTER ELEVEN

Practicing Friendship in the
"Thin Places"

Australian social worker and theologian Lorna Hallahan describes living with disabling conditions as "rabbit hole experiences"—experiences that make people feel like they have fallen down Alice's rabbit hole into a strange and often confusing new world. In Chapter 2, we presented the "rabbit hole experiences" of people hearing their physicians pronounce the diagnosis of dementia for themselves or persons they love. Hallahan goes on to say that long before Lewis Carroll described the adventures of *Alice in Wonderland*, Celtic mythology spoke of "thin places." Often hidden in dense forests, beside streams, the thin places could be frightening and dangerous; they were fraught with suffering but also held opportunities for people to show courage and wisdom. In these thin places, humans felt themselves to be close to the mystery of the holy; they were places of religious ritual and of burial. Hallahan notes that the Celtic word describing the thin place derives from the Latin word *limen*, or, as we generally say today, *threshold*.[1] It is the border between the known and the unknown, the finite and the infinite, the secular and the sacred. Hallahan (2008) writes: "Those of us who intervene in the lives of people in suffering, notably here people living with disability—at times of affliction, loss, grief, illness, and near death—occupy these thin places and how we handle ourselves there is absolutely important" (100).

Although Hallahan was thinking about social workers, clergy, physicians, and others who "intervene" in these thin places, friends accompanying one another on the dementia road meet in thin places, too. They may feel like they have both fallen down the rabbit hole and entered a disorienting new world that can be sometimes terrifying and sometimes delightful. Friends may walk through the thin place as a twosome, but others travel in the company of a community. We explore both approaches in this chapter.

This image of people setting out to journey through the thin place of dementia with their friends recalls the beginnings of so many great adventure tales, in fiction as well as in contemporary video games: you start by consulting a wise person. In this case, the wise persons are those already diagnosed with dementia.

What Do People Want?

The international journal *Dementia* was launched in 2002 to provide a forum for innovative social research and practice related to various forms of progressive forgetfulness. Its editors are committed to inviting persons who have dementia to suggest research topics the journal should address and also to contribute articles for publication alongside the papers by academic researchers. The decision to listen respectfully to persons who have dementia—instead of just talking about them—has resulted in a journal that is different from most in the world of academic publishing. Respected researchers submit their work, but one senses always in reading their articles that, like the editors, they are committed to meeting people in the thin places.

In the second issue of the journal, two persons diagnosed with dementia wrote the introductory guest editorial. Morris Friedell,[2] an American sociology professor before his diagnosis with dementia, and Christine Bryden, an Australian public policy expert before her diagnosis (we mentioned her request for a spiritual director in Chapter 7), titled their editorial "A Word from Two Turtles" (2002). In their essay, they called for more research on how people cope with dementia and the ways that different environments affect coping and daily life. They noted their experience of the limitations of the medical model of dementia, which views them only in terms of their damaged brains; instead, they want their adaptive responses to their brain problems to be emphasized. In other words, their continuing capacity for empathy, curiosity, kindness, and creativity should be included in the research agenda for the coming years. Finally, they stated that they want more researchers to recognize their spirituality as a resource they draw on in living with dementia.

Friedell and Bryden have been leaders in DASNI, the Dementia Advocacy Support Network International (www.dasninternational.org), which began in 2000. The notion of persons who have dementia actively organizing an advocacy group is a twenty-first-century development that many people might find surprising. After all, the public image of dementia is of persons in the advanced stages, usually living in long-term care residences—people far along in the dementia process. However, as we have shown in earlier chapters, more people who have dementia are living full, independent lives in our communities, thanks to the increasing emphasis on early diagnosis and interventions that can slow the progression of cognitive loss. Connecting with other persons similarly diagnosed—persons journeying through "dementia land," as DASNI members call it (Clare, Rowlands, and Quin 2008)—can be a powerful source of strength and support. In addition, these connections can form the basis for advocacy—advocacy for research, changes in public policy, and an end to the stigma associated with dementia.

Organizations like DASNI will undoubtedly grow and spread in coming years. Members of the baby-boom cohort who are comfortable with the use of the Internet for political organizing and social networking will be making their voices heard. Since the founding of DASNI at the turn of the century, organizations like Alzheimer's Disease International, the Alzheimer's Society (Great Britain), and the Alzheimer's Association (United States) have appointed persons diagnosed with dementia to their boards of directors.

Friedell, Bryden, and others have clearly stated what they want from researchers, public policy makers, medical professionals, and others involved with various support services. But what do persons who have dementia say about what they want from their friends? Richard Taylor, a clinical psychologist who is living with dementia, gives us an idea about this in his book *Alzheimer's from the Inside Out* (2007).[3] He complains that friends sometime shout at him, assuming for some reason that forgetfulness is associated with hearing loss. He advises friends not to simplify their speech just because they are talking with him, but rather to be sensitive to whether he understands it. He wants his friends to look him in the eyes, use his name in conversation, share reminiscences without expecting that he will have the same memories, be honest with him, and appreciate the difference between what he says and what he thinks and feels. He writes, "For instance, if I call you 'Mom' or 'Dad,' I am probably not confusing you with my mom or dad; I know they are dead. I may be thinking about the feelings and behaviors I associate with mom and dad. I miss those feelings; I need them. It's just that I so closely associate those feelings with my mom and dad that the words I use become interchangeable when I talk about them. I don't take the time or I can't or won't make the distinction between the people and the feelings" (135).

Most of all, Taylor wants to be treated as a "Thou" and not as an "it." He uses this terminology from the work of Martin Buber throughout his book. For example, in a passage in which he describes the "strange land" of what we are calling the "thin places," he says,

My behavior is treated as something apart from me. "It's not him, it's the disease." Unfortunately, I am both, and to the extent the disease has altered my behavior and thinking, it has altered who I am.

I am no longer who I formerly was. I am no longer like everyone, but there is still a good deal of me left.

My heart aches and I want to shout: "I'm a different Thou, not a quarter It and three quarters Thou." (150–51)

Richard Taylor, Morris Friedell, Christine Bryden, and many other persons living with early-stage dementia and courageously speaking out about their experiences with memory loss agree that they present friends with a challenge. On the one hand, they do not want to be treated differently just because they have difficulty with memory and other aspects of cognition; on the other hand, they recognize that they cannot always track a conversation, sometimes forget what they want to say in the middle of saying it, and repeat themselves (while often reading facial expressions of discomfort on their conversation partners' faces).

Thanks to the drugs that help some people who are in the early stages of dementia, changes in diet and exercise now recommended by some geriatric psychiatrists, and psychosocial interventions like support groups, brain and memory fitness programs, and creative engagement activities, people journeying into "dementia land" are living longer in their communities. Some researchers are starting to report plateauing as a result of early diagnosis, followed by multiple forms of treatment such that some persons with diagnosed dementia may never progress to the point where they can no longer live independently or with a relative. The same can be said for persons described as having mild cognitive impairment (MCI). Despite the evidence some researchers have presented showing a high probability of eventual conversion to Alzheimer's disease, it is important to remember the report on the meta-analysis of forty-one research studies that we discussed in Chapter 1. Its authors concluded that "most people with MCI will not progress to dementia even after 10 years of follow-up" (Mitchell and Shiri-Feshki 2009, 252). This suggests that friends can learn to make accommodations for memory problems and then expect to experience few other changes in the ways they interact. Nevertheless, no research suggests that it is possible to cure Alzheimer's disease and other dementias. Thus, we will continue to have friends who experience the progressive losses typically associated with dementia, losses that eventually mean they will not be able to live like Richard, Morris, and Christine. They will need more daily care than their relatives and friends can provide, which means that they will have to live in community with others with dementia, with most of their care provided by persons being paid (though usually not paid well).

"Make New Friends but Keep the Old"

"One is silver and the other gold." This old song, sung as a three-part round by generations of Girl Scouts, expresses an important prescription for the social relationships of fifth-graders sitting around a campfire. It is just as important for aging persons. As we grow older, we need to be intentional about preserving long-time friendships and about forming new ones, and yet at this time in life, keeping old friends and making new friends becomes more challenging, especially if a move to some form of long-term care is necessary. Given these challenges, it is good to recall Aristotle's description of friendship that we discussed earlier:

> We wish good for our friends and seek to do good on their behalf;
> We want our friends to continue to exist and will do what is in our power to guard
>   and protect them;
> We commit to spending time with our friends;
> We share with our friends common choices and decisions centered in the effort to
>   live virtuous lives; and
> We share in our friends' joys and sorrows. (*Nicomachean Ethics* 9.4.1)

Of course, all of this is much easier said than done. If couples have shared friendships, the death of one member of the couple changes the rhythms and patterns of those friendships. Relocation after retirement separates friends and reduces their face-to-face contact. Various physical problems force friends to give up shared activities. The memory problems and confusion experienced by friends who have dementia mean that new ways of communicating need to be established. None of this is easy. As we have noted, even without any of these challenges, long-time friendships can hit rough patches, which sometimes lead to dissolution of the friendship. These experiences—a partner's death, relocation, physical or mental disability, or strains in a long friendship—have the potential to evoke the kind of fear and anxiety we discussed earlier. What if my mate dies? Does my friend still care about me now that she and her husband have moved to Idaho to be near their children? How would I feel if I had to give up golf like my friend did? What if I am the one diagnosed with dementia? What if the person I thought was my friend no longer wants to be my friend?

Forming new friendships is even more difficult than maintaining vitality in old friendships as the exigencies of aging mount. Making a new friend involves risk, patience, and intentionality. Although occasionally we meet someone for the first time and feel an immediate connection, most of the time friendship requires time to develop and is not a guaranteed outcome. A person in midlife and beyond has accumulated a complex personal story, and it may feel risky to open up that story to a stranger. As we grow older, we tend to become more cautious, not only in how we move through the physical world but also in our negotiations with the social world. Thus, relationships may remain as "acquaintanceships," enjoyable enough, though not as satisfying or meaningful as being with someone who "really knows you." Even acquaintanceships can be demanding, and people may decide they cannot invest themselves in them.

> Betty, who is 76, has been widowed for four years. After her husband died, she moved to an apartment near the home of her son and his wife. She keeps in touch with old friends through email, phone calls, and occasional visits when they "meet in the middle," each driving about an hour for a visit over lunch. After Betty had lived in her apartment about a year, a single woman who appeared to be about her age moved in next door. Betty waited a few weeks and then knocked on her door and introduced herself. She invited the new neighbor to go with her to a program at the Senior Center, and the neighbor seemed happy to do so. Betty thought the woman had a good time and waited for her to reciprocate with a suggestion for another shared activity. The invitation never came. Betty commented to one of her old friends, "Well, I guess she didn't like me," and made no further effort to connect with her neighbor.

Perhaps Betty's neighbor did not want further interaction with Betty. However, the neighbor could be shy and hesitant about contacting Betty, who seemed to know lots of people at the Senior Center. The neighbor might be experiencing some memory problems and has forgotten the trip to the Senior Center, Betty's name, and where she wrote Betty's phone number. There could be hundreds of reasons why Betty's neighbor has not called her, but for Betty, who has felt insecure about relationships throughout her life, it is too psychologically risky to invest any more effort in finding out if a friendship might be possible with the neighbor. That cheerful old Girl Scout song about making new friends holds no hint of how hard this can be.

> George, in his early sixties, was nearing retirement and decided that he needed to start volunteering as a way of giving back and also to find out if it would provide some new role for him once he was no longer working. He heard about a visitation program sponsored by his church that matched people with nursing home residents who were church members. He decided to give it a try and started visiting an elderly man who had multiple physical problems and mild

dementia. Joseph, who was widowed and had no children, seemed happy to have George's company. Because George was still working, he could visit only on weekends, so he started to make a regular practice of going to see Joseph on Sunday afternoons. Joseph tended to tell the same stories over and over—stories of his early years, his experiences in the army, and his life of hard work. The room at the nursing home was warm, and George sometimes felt he might doze off as listened to Joseph repeat his stories, often with the same words he had used the week before. Occasionally, Joseph asked George about what was happening in his life. Over time, George began to feel himself growing close to Joseph, and he discovered that his time with Joseph was deeply relaxing, something he began to look forward to every week.

George began his relationship with Joseph with a sense of obligation. He had taken on a volunteer position with his church's visitation program and was dutiful in fulfilling its expectations. He never imagined that Sunday afternoons with Joseph would become such an important part of his week, or that a forgetful old man in a nursing home could become a friend. This was not a friendship built on a shared history or even on shared interests. And yet, there was reciprocity, although not in the usual sense of the term. Joseph valued George's visits, for he had few other visitors, and most of his contact with people was with the nursing home employees. George came to see his time with Joseph as a gift. It forced him to slow down, turn off his Blackberry, put aside the multitasking that made up the rest of his week, and be "in the moment." Time spent with Joseph felt almost meditative.

Developmental psychologist Robert Kegan would say that George had been "recruited" by Joseph (1982). In other words, somewhat to his surprise, George was drawn into a relationship with an old man who repeated the same stories and was happy to see him every time he walked into his overly warm nursing-home room. George cared about Joseph; Joseph was important to George. When he first began visiting, Joseph had no such feelings; George was just a forgetful old man, rather indistinguishable from all the other forgetful old men at the nursing home. But George came to see Joseph differently; Joseph became a *person* to him. In Kegan's words, "what the eye sees better the heart feels more deeply" (16).

Kegan points out that infants' "cuteness" automatically recruits adults to them. Few adults can resist the allure of a baby's face. This is a biologically based response that is essential for the infant's survival and development. In other words, babies are cute for a reason. But what about old people, especially old people who have moderate to severe memory problems? What characteristics might recruit our attention? As with any relationship that is just beginning, we can learn their names and get to know their faces well enough that they can be recognized. We can look at and into their eyes, even if the eyes gazing back at us cannot see. Kegan writes, "Nowhere does the body have more contours and contrasting shapes than on the face, and nowhere is the contrast greater than the area of the eyes" (17).

Getting to know any person, especially an older person who has progressive forgetfulness, requires patience and the intentionality of repeated contact. One must risk *seeing* the other in the sense of allowing the heart to be moved, rather than merely *looking*. As Kegan says, this can be "dangerous," for it means that we may move into relationship with another person. When we allow ourselves to get close enough to another person, to really *see* that person and be recruited,

> [we] not only increase the likelihood of our being moved; we also run the risk that being moved entails. For we are moved somewhere, and that somewhere is further into life, closer to those we live with. They come to matter more. Seeing better increases our vulnerability to being recruited to the welfare of another. It is our recruitability, as much as our knowledge of what to do once drawn, that makes us of value in our caring for another's development. . . . And why is it so important that we be recruitable? The answer is that a person's life depends (literally in the first few years of life, and in every other way in all the years that follow) on whether he or she moves someone in this way. (16–17)

The common stereotype of the nursing home as a dreary, depressing place is contradicted by the progressive changes occurring in organizations that have adopted the new culture of care we described in Chapter 3.[4] These long-term care residences offer environmental and organizational supports for recruitability; they are communities that can justifiably be described as flourishing. Comfortable public spaces with natural lighting, snacks, and programming that encourages interaction between residents and visitors all can create a place for friendships to grow.

Both parties in these relationships—the person who is living with dementia and the new or old friend who cares—enact the "drama of embrace" that we described in the last chapter. For George, embrace was more than a metaphor. As his visits with Joseph in the nursing home took on more meaning and he sensed their mutual recognition of the importance of the time they spent together, it seemed natural to lean over Joseph's chair when the visit ended to give him a hug.

One might not think of nursing homes as crucibles for new friendships; George certainly had no such idea when he signed up to visit Joseph. And yet, we have repeatedly heard people describe how they have made new friends when they allowed themselves truly to *see* residents, including residents who are living with dementia. Residents may have forgotten the names of family members and friends, along with details about their shared lives, but the human need for meaningful relationships is not affected by the progression of forgetfulness. When asked by sensitive, patient researchers willing to listen to them, people with moderate to severe dementia can describe their awareness of loneliness (Clare et al. 2008a), their sense of dislocation and isolation, and the value they place on continuing friendships as well as new friendships formed in the care facility (Clare et al. 2008b). Although they identified strength and resilience in many residents, overall Linda Clare and her research team found "prominent feelings of loss, isolation, uncertainty, fear, and worthlessness" (717) that were directly tied to "the absence of positive relationships" (718).

What can be done about this? Clare and her colleagues offered seven concrete ideas on how residential homes can ameliorate the sense of isolation and loneliness experienced by persons who have dementia. These recommendations are meant primarily for administrators and staff of these homes, but two can also apply to people like George, who are willing to take the risk of remaining in relationship with old friends—and making new friends—with those who have traveled the dementia road beyond the zone of "early stage." In the next sections, we present specific information on how friends can be a part of the social care that Clare and her colleagues believe must be a part of all care—whether in residential care facilities or in the wider community—of persons who are living with dementia. Before we proceed, however, we need to pause to quote them: "[Provide] more opportunities for conversation with conversational partners who are able to sustain meaningful interaction, and offer basic training in the necessary skills to staff, volunteers, and family members. . . . [Encourage] a sense of community and belonging within the home by facilitating the development of friendships among residents, for example by introducing residents to one another repeatedly and engaging them in group activities, and supporting the development of positive attachments to staff" (Clare et al. 2008b, 718).

Providing Opportunities for Conversation

Conversation is a verbal expression of communication, but communication—the exchange of thoughts and feelings—is not always verbal. In *Navigating the*

Alzheimer's Journey: A Compass for Caregiving (2004), Carol Bowlby Sifton refers to the "first language, the unspoken language of the body" (196). She talks about how difficult it can be to return to the first language because adults have become so focused on verbal communication. Gestures, body positions, facial expressions, and touch can all be forms of communication, although when using first language, we need to be aware of boundaries set by social and cultural heritages. That is, some people may be uncomfortable with touch, and gestures can mean different things in different cultures. Always there must be awareness of the other person's response and willingness to change course if it appears that some form of first-language communication has become distressing. Sifton offers some suggestions for familiar activities of touch that a friend might find comforting: allowing the other to hold on while walking, rubbing in hand cream, gentle massage of the shoulders, and even dancing. She warns that people need to be aware of the fragility of older people's skin and that touch must always be appropriate.

Sifton also addresses spoken communication and begins with the cardinal rule for communication with any older person: remember that this is an adult! Although people often facilely talk about a second infancy, no adult is an infant, and to behave as if the person is an infant is highly insulting and dehumanizing. One can, however, be intentional about speaking positively, using short sentences, and providing what Sifton calls "orienting cues" (216). That is, employing a casual conversational style, friends can say their names and mention something immediate about the day. "Hi, Mary. I'm your friend Jessie and I've stopped by for a little visit today. It sure is cold on this blustery November day." Often, one finds that people who have dementia display "astonishingly adept social manners" (Hellebrandt 1978, 68), for the "social graces" they learned in their youth have been well practiced. Thus, Mary, not recognizing her friend Jessie, might reply, "Oh, hello. How are you today?" And thus a conversation is begun.

The conversation should not then turn into a game of twenty questions. It can meander into many different topics, and it really does not matter if the person with memory problems is telling a story accurately. After all, cognitive psychologists have long known that memory is reconstructive. Persons who have no signs of progressive forgetfulness do not recall events as if they are running mental documentary films and describing what they see. Instead of viewing the conversation as reminiscence, which accurately relates events from the past, one can think of it as storytelling. Just as much meaning—perhaps more—is communicated through storytelling than through reporting.

Storytelling can be enhanced in a variety of ways. For example, sometimes friends look through photo albums together. They may listen to music they both enjoy and then talk about what they associate with it. Depending on the friend's interests, certain books might captivate them. For example, in a creative engagement group held at our county nursing home, one man with advanced dementia focused full attention on creating clay forms for about a half hour, and for the rest of the time, with a volunteer, he intently paged through a book of beautiful photographs of clay pots from cultures around the world. He had entered his "joy zone."

People often wonder what they can *do* with their friends who have dementia. Much of this depends on the level of forgetfulness and other problems the person might have (e.g., with mobility). But, it also depends on who they are as persons and the things that have brought pleasure and meaning in the past. Helping a person continue to be engaged with some kind of hobby can add enjoyment to the day. One care partner once told us that she wished that her husband had just one friend who would take him to a place by a local lake where he had fished for many years. Sadly, no one had stepped up to do that, and she felt reluctant to ask. Some people might want to play an old familiar game together, while others just enjoy sitting and chatting.

Sometimes, conversations with friends who have dementia may wander into what some might describe as nonsense, and this is the time it is especially important to "listen with the third ear," as psychoanalyst Theodor Reik (1948) called it. Of course, the friend is not attending to the subtexts of the conversation and the nonverbal cues of body position and vocal expression in order to psychoanalyze the other. Rather, this kind of listening reflects a willingness to set aside expectations about linear conversation, which proceeds neatly from one point to another. After all, what conversation between friends without memory loss actually does this? When one allows oneself to listen like this, one can hear remarkably insightful, even poetic, statements. One of our favorites came from a woman who quietly said, "My foot is crying" to describe the pain she felt. If we had not been listening carefully to her, or if we had immediately dismissed this as an irrational statement, the poetry of that moment would have been lost.

Another way of describing this kind of communication is to call it "relational mindfulness" (McFadden 2008). Psychologists describe mindfulness in terms of focused attention—being in the moment. While noting its ancient roots in meditative practices, they are now peering into the brain via various imaging technologies to see why mindfulness seems to be associated with stress reduction and health promotion. This type of mindfulness often occurs in solitude (unless, of course, you have your head in a large MRI magnet, with technicians hovering about). Sometimes, groups undertake mindfulness exercises, as when they sit together, listening to someone lead them through a guided-imagery exercise. Relational mindfulness, on the other hand, refers to the experience of connecting with another person without allowing attention to be drawn away to one's own personal projects. George learned to practice relational mindfulness with Joseph. Even though he had heard Joseph's tales of his early life over and over, he disciplined himself not to allow his mind to wander and to enter into the moment of the conversation as if it was the first time he had heard Joseph's story.

When visiting with a friend who has memory loss, people need to be alert for signs of fatigue, to regulate as much as possible the immediate environment to reduce distractions, and to be comfortable with silence. This is hard for many people to do, but it can be a part of mindfulness discipline that friends can acquire. Whether the conversation takes place in someone's private home, a public place like a coffee shop, or at a long-term care residence, it is important to be sensitive to fatigue and the rhythms of the day. For example, persons who are living with moderate to severe dementia can experience what has come to be called "sundowning"—an increase in agitation and confusion in the late afternoon and into the evening hours (Nowak and Davis 2007). Care partners are the best source of insight into the times of day when a visit with a friend would be most welcomed; they are good at describing activity patterns and their variability during the day (Chung, Ellis-Hill, and Coleman 2008). Distractions like a television or people entering and leaving the room can also interrupt the flow of conversation. Because persons who have dementia may also have problems with hearing and vision, their friends should be sensitive to these additional challenges to communication.

Communication does not always have to be conversational. One can sit quietly with a friend and observe the world outside a window, watch the movements of fish or birds (many long-term care residences now have fish tanks and aviaries), or listen to music. If one spends time in silence with a friend, there should still be intentionality about relating to the friend: gesture toward a child riding by outside on a bicycle or the bird scrabbling for seed, or note the rhythm of the music with hand movements.[5]

Encouraging a Sense of Community

In their paper that noted the loneliness of people who are living with dementia, Clare et al. (2008b) focused on those with moderate to severe dementia who had moved into residential care. They urged staff members to be intentional about creating a sense of community among residents by nurturing residents' positive interactions with one another and with the staff. In communities, people call one another by their preferred names; persons who have dementia might forget these names, so intentional community building requires that names be repeated as a normal part of social life. In the kind of community Clare and colleagues envision, the staff know important details about residents' identities and share information about themselves appropriately (e.g., "You're wearing blue today, my favorite color!" not "I had a big fight with my boyfriend last night and threw him out").

Friends can help to encourage a sense of community, both for persons living in residential care as well as for individuals—some of whom are still in the early stages of progressive forgetfulness—who live alone or with family members. This community building can evolve informally, and it can also be a part of participation in structured activities, both in the wider community and in residential care.

Mary's long-time friend Sarah had progressed in forgetfulness to the point that her family decided she needed full-time residential care. At first, Mary was uncomfortable about visiting Sarah at Garden View, for she had bad memories of nursing homes from her younger years, when her grandmother had lived in one. However, she soon discovered that Sarah's new residence was a different kind of place, a place where people lived in small households, each of which had a public living room. The households (consisting of private rooms for eleven persons) were organized into neighborhoods (a combination of three households), and each neighborhood had its own public area, where residents often gathered. Garden View also had a large community room attached to an area organized like a café. Residents could hang out there together, sipping beverages purchased from a vending machine, eating popcorn made every afternoon, and most important, interacting with one another. This was definitely not her grandmother's nursing home! Mary soon came to look forward to her visits with Sarah. She chatted with Sarah but also drew other residents into the conversation. Regardless of where she and Sarah sat for their visit, Mary was intentional about including other residents, calling them by name, and reintroducing them to Sarah. Thus, supported by architecture and interior design that encouraged interpersonal interaction, and motivated by her personal knowledge of Sarah's social nature, Mary became a community builder.

Mary was able to assist in building community with her old friend Sarah for several reasons. Because she visited Sarah on a regular basis (usually once a week), she became familiar and comfortable with the physical and social environment where Sarah lived. Garden View's design made social interaction easy and pleasant. Despite her loyalty to Sarah, Mary might not have been as apt to visit regularly if Sarah lived in a place like the one her grandmother had spent her last years in, a nursing home with long dark halls, whose only community space was the dining area, which always had a lingering odor of overcooked meat and vegetables. Finally, Mary's personality was outgoing and she enjoyed people. Thus, she felt comfortable getting to know other residents and sharing her time with Sarah with them. This demonstrates the important interaction of personal and environmental characteristics that support the enhancement of a sense of community.

A place like the one where Sarah lives invites informal community building. It vividly reminds us that we need new language for talking about this kind of residential living, for to say that Sarah is institutionalized completely ignores the rich possibilities for social interaction available at Garden View. Paradoxically, it may be easier for people who are living with dementia to experience a sense of a shared life at a place like Garden View than if they still reside "in the community." In other words, so-called community-dwelling elders can be more socially isolated and thus offer friends a greater challenge to keep them engaged with other people.

Bill, who has been retired for a decade, has been a member of his local Kiwanis Club for more than thirty-five years. It meets weekly over the noon hour at a local restaurant. Although new people have joined the club, Bill usually sits at a table with people he has known a long time. A few months ago, it finally dawned on Bill that he had not seen or heard from his friend Jim for a while. He called Jim's home and, in a conversation with Jim's wife, Agnes, learned that Jim had been diagnosed with early-stage Alzheimer's disease and was no longer able to drive. Agnes described how he seemed to be getting along pretty well, although she was feeling increasingly stressed and isolated as she felt her own social world shrinking because she felt she had to spend most of her time with Jim. Bill offered to start taking Jim to the Kiwanis Club meetings. At first, Agnes wasn't sure she wanted Bill to do this; she worried that Jim might embarrass himself by spilling food or not keeping up with the conversation. Bill was sensitive to her concerns and kept insisting that Jim would be fine and that he would make sure Jim was welcomed and made comfortable among their group of old friends. Agnes trusted Bill and conceded that she relished being able to count on having two hours a week to do errands, have lunch with her own friends, or just sit and sew.

Bill has made a commitment to help Jim remain engaged in his community. It requires effort, not only to pick Jim up and take him home after the Kiwanis gathering but also to make sure Jim knows the people sitting at the table and is included in the conversation. Bill needs to pay attention to Jim's needs, like making sure they stop in the bathroom before and after lunch. He has to be sure that Jim can manage the food served that day and that he can maneuver in and out of the car and into the restaurant. It would undoubtedly be much easier for Bill just to go to the meetings by himself, but he is loyal to his friend and understands how important it is for Jim to continue to feel embraced by this particular community.

Bill and Mary are informally building community with and for their friends who have dementia. This kind of activity can also occur with organized settings that usually are labeled as "programs" for persons who have dementia. For example, Mary might volunteer to assist with a creative engagement group that Sarah attends, perhaps one that employs the Time*Slips* creative storytelling method developed by Anne Basting (2009). There are many types of creative engagement programs being integrated into the daily life of residential care homes and adult day programs. Their primary goals are to encourage individual expression by persons who often lack opportunities or capacity to communicate and also to build and strengthen social connections (McFadden and Basting 2010). These programs are structured carefully to achieve the latter goal by beginning and ending in rituals of greeting and parting. Leaders (often paid staff) and volunteers move around the circle of participants, greeting everyone by name and introducing persons to one another. When the session ends, participants are thanked individually for their participation and contribution to the group's experience of creative engagement. Using the Time*Slips* method, persons who have dementia create a story together. Other approaches, such as Memories in the Making™, involve individuals working on a personal project (painting, in the case of Memories), but there is always a social element, not just in the greeting and parting rituals, but also when each person shares with the group what he or she has created.

Once persons embrace the idea of building community to include their friends who have dementia, many possible venues emerge. For example, most senior centers offer a vast array of opportunities for recreation, learning, and travel. However, participants who have not experienced memory loss may initially resist including individuals who have progressive forgetfulness. This is an occasion when people who have learned to allow compassion to overrule fear and anxiety can act as important role models in community building. Staff support for inclusion is also important.

Another, more formally structured setting for building community can be found in religious worship services, whether at a residential care home or in a church, synagogue, temple, or mosque. Worship at a residential care home can be a meaningful experience, especially when family members and friends accept the role of being active participants in the worshipping community, one that includes but reaches beyond the person they know who resides in the care home. Together, young and old, mentally fit and cognitively disabled persons sing, pray, listen to the reading of sacred texts, participate in religious rituals, and in some settings, move around to greet one another in a state of relational mindfulness, a practice sometimes called "passing the peace."

Outside of residential care, people can make sure their friends who have dementia can attend worship and feel welcome when they do. This might require the congregation to develop special worship programs for individuals with memory loss if the regular worship service is too loud, wordy, or fast paced.[6] After all, congregations never seem to object to providing services appropriate for children, so why should they not do the same for persons who have dementia?

John Swinton (2000) suggested that congregations should appoint people to be dementia advocates. He defines a dual role for an advocate: "to defend and to comfort" (174). The dementia advocate in a congregation would stand firm against stigmatization and assumptions that persons with memory loss cannot (or should not) participate in the life of the congregation. The advocate would comfort persons with the diagnosis and their families who feel excluded and would work to overcome barriers to inclusion. In other words, the dementia advocate would take on a leadership role in community building. Other community organizations, like senior centers, service clubs, and recreation centers, could also benefit from people adopting the role of the dementia advocate.

In the early stages of dementia, persons with the diagnosis can be advocates alongside their friends, working to create and secure meaningful community connections and acceptance of persons who have dementia. We already can observe this happening as people bravely declare that they have stepped onto the dementia road and need to be treated as valued members of their communities. Essentially, they are stating that despite their cognitive state, they possess the status, duties, and rights of *citizens*, acting not only out of concern for their own personal well-being but also to secure respect for all who share their diagnosis. In other words, people like Richard Taylor, Morris Friedell, and Christine Bryden, whom we met at the beginning of this chapter, are claiming the role of active citizens and not tragic victims of a disease (Bartlett and O'Connor 2007).[7]

The notion of the citizenship of persons who have dementia leads to our last point about what it means to create a vital sense of community in which people have the opportunity to be meaningfully engaged with one another. Community is more than knowing people's names and something about one another's identity, personal history, and interests. It is more than just "hanging out" together, important as that kind of informal socializing can be. Although community connections can be strengthened through various intentional programs like the ones we have mentioned here, there is still something missing in this discussion. In flourishing communities, people work together to secure meaningful lives not just for themselves but for other persons, too. As we said in previous chapters, in flourishing communities people experience a sense of mutual obligation, knowing that we all live with vulnerability. Up until the last stages of dementia, people can express that mutuality through serving others. Friends can help make this happen.

Being of Service to Others

In an earlier chapter, we stated that faith communities honor persons who have dementia by continuing to expect them to fulfill their obligations to show love to others. What generally gets labeled as "service" or "voluntarism" does not have to be motivated by religious faith or take place within a religious environment. Today, many people are talking about how the baby-boom generation might respond to the call to volunteer once their careers wind down. However, descriptions of encore careers (paid or volunteer activities after retirement from the primary career) do not acknowledge how people living with memory loss might participate.

Several studies indicate that persons who have dementia very much want to be included in the emerging new opportunities for older adult community service. For example, in a paper describing how they created the "Dementia Quality of Life Instrument," Meryl Brod and colleagues related how they conducted focus groups with people in the early stages of memory loss to learn what contributed to their feelings of good life quality. Among other things, they noted that their participants "expressed the desire to be of more service to their community and family, and expressed pain at not having an opportunity to contribute something of worth to others" (Brod et al. 1999, 33). In the revised edition of her influential book *Speaking Our Minds*, Lisa Snyder (2009) quoted a retired psychologist who had Alzheimer's disease and stated this desire: "I'd like to help people find meaning instead of just sitting home and disappearing. I would like to be part of something where I belong and it has meaning to me" (161). One of the seven people featured in Snyder's book described what his experiences at a weekly gathering of people with mild to moderate memory loss meant to him.[8] He said, "The word *Alzheimer* is never mentioned, and we laugh a lot during the whole four hours. We discuss news of the day, do calisthenics, and then we work on a community service project" (Snyder 2009, 50).

Opportunities for people who are living with dementia to be of service to others are proliferating, although they have not received as much publicity as programs like Civic Ventures (www.civicventures.org), a nonprofit think tank that promotes encore careers. One of the best-known volunteer programs for people who have dementia is the Intergenerational School (TIS: www.tisonline.org), founded by Peter and Cathy Whitehouse, in Cleveland, Ohio. Peter Whitehouse, a geriatrician and researcher who has written extensively about dementia, urges his patients to find ways to volunteer in their communities. TIS brings children together with older people, including individuals diagnosed with Alzheimer's and other dementias, for reading, mentoring, and story-sharing. Other programs of TIS involve gardening, arts projects, and using computers (Whitehouse and George 2008).

In Chicago, at the Alzheimer's Family Care Center (an adult day service), many participants recall a long history of formal voluntarism, often through their churches or synagogues, and informal service to neighbors and people in their communities. Through a program developed by the Family Care Center, participants sort clothes for the Salvation Army, provide activities for children living at a domestic abuse shelter, create materials for children's learning at a museum, help students with their reading, and work with nonprofit organizations to prepare mailings. When she led a focus group with participants to learn more about their experience, Jane Stansell, the director of the center, learned that volunteering helped them feel competent, provided a sense of meaning, and contributed to their feelings of well-being (Stansell 2002).

Individuals committed to creating lives of meaning and purpose for their friends who have dementia can encourage community organizations to welcome various kinds of voluntarism by persons living with memory loss. They can help to inform organizations about their friends' desire to feel useful and helpful to others and about the accommodations that might need to be made due to the memory difficulties. Friends could volunteer alongside their friends who have dementia, being watchful for their safety and levels of stamina and strength.

Progressive long-term care residences usually welcome the participation of community members, who either are already friends of residents or who become friends through regular interaction with them. Often this takes the form of one-to-one visitation, but we think that this model needs to be expanded to include community building, not only through creative engagement programs such as we described earlier, but also through organized service projects. As Stansell learned, people who are living with dementia recall various forms of service from the past. Friends of persons who have dementia could advocate for the formation of service clubs at long-term care residences as a way of building community and providing the opportunity to preserve a sense of meaning and purpose. In this way, together they can create flourishing communities.

What Happens after We Say "Hello" in the Thin Places?

In a blog post to Alzheimer's Daily News (www.alznews.org), Richard Taylor wrote on April 9, 2008, that a diagnosis of Alzheimer's disease should mean "hello" and not "good-bye." He described the feeling of fading away that is reinforced by others who hear about the diagnosis and start to withdraw. Acutely aware of his own problems, which he sometimes finds embarrassing, he nevertheless boldly asserted, "I'm still me!" He continued: "Isn't it time others who don't live with the diagnosis focus their energies on understanding, appreciating, supporting, enabling those of us who do live with diagnosis? . . . I, and I honestly believe every other person living with dementia, need to hear, feel, and be supported by saying 'Hello!' "

The question this chapter has addressed is what friends might do after they say "hello"—after they make the commitment to stay in friendship or to form a new friendship in the place where the world of memory loss and memory retention meet. This place can be both treacherous and transcendent. It is a new place, wrought by increased life expectancy and various psychosocial and pharmacological treatments that retard—but do not reverse or halt—the progress of dementia. It is a place fraught with challenges and opportunities, and it is a place where more and more of us will be meeting in this new time of dementia.

After we say "hello," we can choose to be in relationship with one another, to listen to one another, and together, to build flourishing communities that give us all a heightened sense of meaning and purpose. We close this chapter with a quote from an article by sociologist Karen Lyman. In this piece, she wrote about how people who have Alzheimer's disease create meaning. "Alzheimer's disease requires living courageously in a brave new world, not simply a world of 'deficits' and 'losses,' but one that includes a new career for survivors: the daily work of recreating meaning and re-affirming the changed self" (Lyman 1998, 56). We agree with Lyman, but we would add that this daily work needs to be done in the company of others—people who have made the commitment to be friends in the thin places.

CHAPTER TWELVE

Memory, Forgetting, and the Present Time

Do not cast me off in the time of old age; Do not forsake me when
my strength is spent.

Psalm 71:9

Anne Basting (2009) argues that our fear of memory loss is greater than it needs
to be because memory is the collective possession of the communities in which
we participate. Although most scientists and geriatricians believe that there are
significant differences between the memory losses associated with so-called
healthy aging and those associated with dementia, all persons are continuously
losing memories, a process that accelerates with aging. Losing memories—
forgetting—is not just inevitable, it is essential to our emotional health. As related in the famous case study by the Russian psychologist A. R. Luria (1968/
1987), a person who has an exceptional memory for every small detail cannot perform the mental functions necessary for grasping generalities, figurative thinking, and abstractions. In other words, we *need* to forget certain particularities—to
clear them away from consciousness—so we can contemplate the meaning of
large, complex, multifaceted ideas.

In Chapter 10, we described Miroslav Volf's images of the "drama of embrace."
Volf (1996) argues that relationships, whether between individuals or societies,
cannot be sustained without mutual forgiveness and that genuine forgiveness
necessarily entails a kind of forgetting. We must let go of the real or imagined
wrong we have suffered and regard it as if it had never occurred or we cannot
succeed in reinvesting essential trust in that relationship. Both individuals and
societies must overcome fear before they can "forgive and forget" because there
is undeniable risk in forgetting. If we forget the offense committed against us,
we leave ourselves vulnerable to suffering a similar offense in the future. By
remembering the wrongs done to us, we remain vigilant and suspicious, thereby
convincing ourselves that we are safe. But the price we pay for such security is
high. We will live with constant anxiety and mistrust and, in the case of wrongs
one society or nation has perpetrated on another, we will school new generations in fear, even hatred. If we cannot forget the wrongs done to us by others we

cannot genuinely forgive, and without forgiveness important relationships cannot be renewed or sustained. The relationships with others that define our selfhood are dependent on our ability and willingness to forget.

Discussion is now developing about the costs of the Internet's inability to "forget." Emails containing confidential information continue to exist on distant servers even after deletion. Arrest records that have been legally expunged remain available to prospective employers through archived newspaper articles. Some fear that that the permanence of information on the Internet is rapidly becoming a barrier to the proper functioning of society because it does not permit us to forget things that are best forgotten.

All this is to say that remembering and forgetting are equally essential to emotional health, relationships with others, and a workable society. We do not wish to minimize the real challenges that come with the progressive memory loss that accompanies dementia, but rather to argue that we need to think of remembering and forgetting in corporate as well as individual terms and that some forms of forgetting are not only valuable but essential to individual and societal well-being. Possession of excellent memory abilities is generally considered a blessing, but it may also become a curse. The memory loss associated with dementia does not stand in contrast to normative expectations that everything is, or should be, remembered. Rather, it falls at one end of a continuum of remembering and forgetting.

It is the role of friends and communities to preserve the valuable and desirable memories that an individual may lose through accident, disease, or the normal process of aging and to continue to include that individual in the recollection of the important stories of the lives we have shared together. In a related way, friends, families, and communities also need to be able to forget. We have seen too many families split by disputes over the care of an elder diagnosed with dementia who has forgotten the misdeeds and hurtful behaviors of the past but whose adult children cannot forget. People may speak facilely about time healing all wounds, but we know that this is not necessarily true. Paradoxically, however, the illness of dementia can produce the healing of relationships when old hurts are set aside—perhaps even forgotten—and loving connections are experienced in the present moment.

Friendship and Time

No community can flourish unless all of its members, including those who are most vulnerable, also flourish. Many communities have already discovered that in expanding the practice of hospitality to embrace persons who have physical disabilities or cognitive limitations they have made the life of the community richer for all who participate. We do not mean simply that they experience the warm glow of knowing they are doing the right thing but that they benefit from the rich array of gifts these participants bring to community life and from the valuable lessons they teach. In many cases they are able to teach others in community to live more fully in the immediate moment—taking time to be present to a friend who may speak slowly or with difficulty and finding that this friend in turn is present to them in ways that make their own lives more joyous and complete. A hospitable community is one in which time is allowed to move a bit more slowly, as frenetic preoccupation with productivity is mitigated by the simple pleasure of being in caring relationship with one another.

> Fred's cerebral palsy necessitates his using a wheelchair and makes simple motor tasks a significant challenge. He must work hard to enunciate words, and even those who regularly interact with him must sometimes ask him to repeat what he says. He works twenty hours each week in the human resources department of a large not-for-profit corporation, laboriously entering data on a specially equipped computer. Each Monday morning the human resources team gathers to share current concerns and activities, with each person in turn providing an update of his or her activities. When it is Fred's turn to speak, the other members of the team concentrate intently on his words, with those most attuned to his speech repeating the occasional word for clarification. Time slows as ten busy people attend to what Fred has to say (which often concludes with an evaluation of the most recent performance by the Green Bay Packers). One Monday, when Fred was absent from work, a team member asked the group, "so who is going to force us to slow down this morning and remember why we do what we do?"

Certainly there are persons traveling the early miles of the dementia road in workplace environments, but those who have journeyed a greater distance are not as likely to be found there. But there are many other communal settings—restaurants, coffee shops, stores, museums, concert halls, bowling alleys, farmers markets, fairs, congregations—where hospitality can be readily extended to include persons who have dementia. The greatest barrier to such hospitality is the manner in which we have allowed ourselves to view dementia as somehow different from and more threatening than other human limitations. This is not true in all cultures. One of us was describing the themes of this book to a woman who grew up in Taiwan before attending medical school in the United States. "I did not realize until I got to medical school that my grandfather had

Alzheimer's," she reflected. "He changed as he got older, but to us, he was still just Grandfather."

At one time in our nation's history, persons who had physical or cognitive disabilities were commonly removed from their families (often placed in institutions in remote locales), while older people who had "a touch of senility" remained active in their communities. This pattern has long since been reversed. One wonders if the fear of aging itself plays some role in the stigmatization of dementia in our time. In the person who has dementia, we see a possible version of our own future in a way we do not in the person who has a congenital disability.

We suggested in Chapter 9 that congregations provide settings in which persons can be schooled in hospitality and friendship. This is not to say that congregations are the only settings in which this may occur. For example, aging-in-place initiatives have given us the term *NORC* (naturally occurring retirement community) to describe apartment buildings or neighborhoods in which the majority of residents are older persons.[1] Once a NORC is recognized as such,[2] a variety of programs can be offered by both governmental and private agencies to bring needed services to the neighborhood and build structures of mutual support, ideally incorporating younger as well as older residents. Communities where friendship and hospitality are practiced can also break forth in many other settings, ranging from barbershops to restaurants and taverns. For example, a coffee shop on Cape Cod has evolved into an informal community center. An article in the *New York Times* described a man—the primary caregiver for a wife who has Alzheimer's disease—who visits the coffee shop each day for a cup of tea and a bit of respite care.[3] Community is wherever we find it or create it.

An example of the intentional creation of communities for mutual support can be found in the small but growing co-housing movement in which residents own their own homes but commit to sharing certain facilities (gardens, guest quarters, laundry room, etc.) and eating several meals a week together.[4] Most co-housing communities encourage diversity of age, income, race, and cognitive and physical abilities, and they center their life in a commitment to friendship and hospitality. But short of such a major lifestyle commitment, congregations remain one of the few settings that bring together a diverse community of persons, including those of different age cohorts, committed to the practices of friendship and hospitality. They stand in a unique position to serve as laboratories for exploring new ways to honor, value, and include persons traveling the dementia road. Thus, to extend the metaphor, they could provide a roadmap for the wider society.

Among other things, congregations might mount a challenge to the wider society's understanding of the nature of time and the manner in which it is to be used. We live with the paradox of ever higher expectations for productivity and the attendant frantic pace of activity, while at the same time we are spending more time watching television than ever (more than four hours per day on average, a number that increases as we grow older, according to Nielsen).[5] For many people, time is spent either working at maximum capacity or recovering from the stress of the workday by zoning out in front of the television, leaving little opportunity for experiencing the goodness of life through friendships and the practices of community.

Congregations are settings in which we can learn to understand time as something other than the too-rapid passing of hours and minutes. To employ the Greek terms, business and commerce take place within *chronos* time, the linear passage of time defined by appointment calendars, goals, and deadlines. If chronos is the horizontal dimension of time passing by, then *kairos* time is the vertical dimension, which is experienced in the present moment, when we become so engaged in immediate experience that we are not even conscious of the passage of time.[6] The Zen koan "The worker is hidden in the workshop" speaks of kairos time: the worker is so thoroughly centered in the task at hand that there is no awareness time's passing, no distinction between the one who works and the work that is being performed. Kairos time is "replete with meaning" (McFadden and Thibault 2001, 231) for individuals and for their collectivities.

Friendship unfolds within kairos time. We meet our friend for coffee, speak of this and that, and bask in the pleasure of each other's company until one person glances at her watch in alarm: "My goodness! Where did the time go?" Chronos time is essential to keep organizations running on schedule, while kairos time is equally essential for individuals and communities to flourish and enjoy the goodness of life together.

Considered strictly in medical terms, the journey into dementia unfolds within linear, chronos time. The disease progresses through various stages, which can be evaluated and quantified. "Your father is clearly in stage two now." "Your wife is moving into the fourth stage, and it is time [chronos] to think about moving her into the memory-care unit." But that journey is also about moving from preoccupation with chronos to the immediate experience of kairos, as the person who has progressive forgetfulness becomes less oriented to calendars and schedules and more focused on living in the present moment. All friendships of depth take place within kairos time, but this is particularly true when one friend has dementia.

Even as friendships are lived within kairos time, the life of community draws us into kairos as well. We shop at the supermarket in chronos time, methodically moving through aisles and filling the cart until the task is accomplished, as quickly and efficiently as possible. But when we visit the farmer's market, we enter kairos time. We chat with the merchants, visit with friends, and get drawn into conversations with strangers—the task becomes secondary to the shared experience of community.

Congregations, like a farmer's market, should be settings in which we appreciate the gift of kairos time, being fully present to one another and open to the gifts and joys the moment may offer us. If, as we have argued in Chapter 9, congregations are called to be "schools for subversive friendship," they must be settings in which persons learn to appreciate the gift of kairos time and the manner in which it allows us to be mindfully present to one another.

Western society has long been focused on finding a cure—a vaccine, a pill, a "magic bullet"—for various diseases and conditions, and in many cases it has been successful in that effort. Sometimes the search for a cure is presented in alarmist, chronos-time terms (especially in fundraising letters) as a "race against the clock to beat this dreaded disease." But there is scant evidence that dementia is a disease that can be traced to a single, curable causal agent. Abhilash Desai,[7] a respected geriatric psychiatrist, argues that we do have a magic bullet that can have significant impact on both the incidence and severity of dementia, but it lacks the convenience of a pill taken daily. It includes vigorous daily exercise, proper attention to diet and nutrition, a strong social support system, giving and receiving love and affection, finding joy and laughter in the pleasures of each day, and being grounded in a strong spiritual center. This is not a prescription tailored for a culture accustomed to quick fixes, but it is one with the potential to create better and more fulfilled lives. Dementia is a condition that must be treated in kairos time as well as in chronos time. It is not the disease of an individual, but a circumstance experienced within a life that is lived in the midst of friends and community.

The *New York Times* ethical advice columnist Randy Cohen was asked this question concerning the obligation of friends to include a man who has Alzheimer's disease in their social activities: "For 25 years we have enjoyed a regular poker game. Tragically, a longtime participant has been stricken with Alzheimer's, to the degree that the game is no longer enjoyable for the rest of us. We hoped he would decide not to play or to join us just for the pregame dinner, but he hasn't. May we ask him or his wife if he would do so?"[8]

Such awkward dilemmas will become more common as greater numbers of persons reach old age, and some journey into dementia. Poker, like many recreational activities, includes elements of both kairos and chronos time. It represents an evening set apart from life's demands so that good friends can enjoy one another's company, which speaks of kairos. But the game itself unfolds in chronos time, as each player in turn plays a hand. It is a game of strategy that makes significant cognitive demands (knowing when to hold, when to fold, and when to bluff) on its participants. It is against this backdrop of linear, strategic play (chronos) that the joy and laughter of friends being present to one another (kairos) unfolds.

In posing their question to Mr. Cohen, the friends are admitting their anxiety about naming "the elephant in the room" directly to their friend or his wife. They have been passively waiting for the situation to resolve itself—for the friend to remove himself from their circle. Commendably, they clearly take the obligation of friendship seriously. They wish to continue including this friend in their ongoing circle of companionship, but a primary form that companionship has taken for many years has become unworkable for all of them. Dementia is experienced not just by an individual, but by a community, and the community is required to negotiate a path that will allow this cherished friend to be included and valued in a manner that works for everyone. Cohen offered a thoughtful response:

> You are of course entitled to your biweekly poker game—I believe that's in the Constitution—and you admirably seek to reconcile that right with the duties of friendship, among which kindness is paramount.
>
> Begin by talking to your friend's wife and seeking her advice: she is surely aware of his condition. She might like the idea of his joining you for dinner but skipping the game. Perhaps she will suggest other ways to reconfigure your gatherings and how most gently to let your friend know of your plans and your affection for him.

All of us will likely face circumstances in which we need to find creative, loving ways to "reconfigure our gatherings." Cohen is certainly correct to argue that the friend's wife needs to be a part of this effort, but we wish he had not seemingly dismissed out of hand the possibility that the friend himself could directly contribute to this effort. Is it not likely that he has, at least at times, been aware that his participation has become challenging for himself and for his friends? Linda Clare's (2003) interviews with persons with early-stage Alzheimer's disease showed that they were aware of their memory problems, although they differed in how they responded, with some being willing to face their difficulties directly, and others being more committed to maintaining continuity with their images of themselves before the onset of memory problems.

Fear and awkwardness can prevent us from addressing these matters with a friend in the early stages of dementia, which is when they should be discussed. Perhaps the conversation could begin like this:

> We have been friends for a long time and will always be friends, and friends need to be honest with each other. Your memory is not what it used to be, and I have the sense that this has made our weekly games more difficult for you. Sometimes it makes it more difficult for the rest of us as well. What can we do differently that will make our evenings as enjoyable for all of us as they have always been?

There might be a number of potential solutions to explore. Perhaps the friend could attend but play only a few hands of poker. Perhaps he could partner with another player. And, if his dementia progresses to the point where this is no longer possible, he could share in the dinner but skip the game. The group could make time for additional activities—visiting a museum together, for example—that are more workable for the one who has dementia.

It requires creativity to reconfigure the gatherings of friends when dementia enters their circle. But the alternative—ignoring the issue until the friend withdraws (or is withdrawn by a family member)—bespeaks fear rather than friendship. Our circles of friendship will need to be reconfigured multiple times as we age together, for change is inevitable in the aging journey. Death or geographic moves will cause cherished friends of many years to leave our "convoy," and new friends will join us along the way. The activities that we share will change as our interests do or as we face new limitations. Dementia is but one of many changes in life's experience that requires such reconfiguration. Friendship, like love, will always find a way.

We now have more than a decade of research documenting that, if the poker player's friends make accommodations so they can continue to include him in their games, then his dementia might not progress so quickly (Bassuk, Glass, and Berkman 1999; Bennett et al. 2006; Fratiglioni, Paillard-Borg, and Winblad 2004; McFadden and Basting 2010). Moreover, this research indicates that if they continue with their games, they may be less likely to develop forgetfulness. In other words, social connectedness may protect against memory loss, and if memory loss is present, having a strong social network can reduce the disability created by the forgetfulness. This message appears throughout David Snowden's remarkable story of the School Sisters of Notre Dame, elderly nuns who agreed to undergo regular cognitive testing and to donate their brains "to science" upon death. Snowden (2001) believed that their lives in religious community protected them by offering intellectual stimulation (after all, many were life-long professional teachers), a healthy diet, and regular exercise (gardening, working in the laundry, cooking for the group) and also that they received some neuroprotection from living among persons who cared deeply for one another. Those sisters whose journeys did take them into dementia continued to be included in community, which meant, above all, regular practices of devotion and worship.

Vulnerability and Strength

In tracing the cultural history of aging in America, Thomas R. Cole (1992) argues that the dramatic contrast between "good aging" and "bad aging" first arose in the Victorian era. For the Victorians, "good" old age was marked by health, prosperity, virtue, and self-reliance, while "bad" old age was defined by sickness, sin, dependency, and premature death. This was very much in keeping with Victorian ideals, in which prosperity, vigor, and self-control were associated with moral virtue, an association that persists into our own era. Cole notes that before 1800 a more balanced and integrated view of aging, largely shaped by Calvinist thought, predominated. Calvinism, with its understanding of human nature as "utterly depraved," saw in the physical and cognitive decay accompanying aging the inevitable consequence of humanity's fallen nature as well as an opportunity for the grace of God to be revealed. "God's grace did not alter the signs of our physical decay, it transformed their meaning. With the tested and refined piety of old age came the strength and courage to face one's condition openly and to fulfill final obligations" (231).

However, within the Victorian mindset, so centered in the importance of self-control, the losses associated with aging took on a more threatening aspect. "The decaying body in old age, a constant reminder of the limits of self-control, came to signify precisely what bourgeois culture hoped to avoid: dependence, disease, failure and sin" (231).

Piety is not a word much used by even the religiously devout in our time, but the traits commonly associated with piety—wisdom, humility, gratitude—are still counted among the virtues many would wish to embody in their later years. Cole is correct to note that these virtues are often born of being "tested and refined" by experiences accumulated over time, particularly experiences of suffering and loss. The Victorian dichotomizing of success versus failure, prosperity versus poverty, and strength versus weakness made suffering a temporary aberration to be stoically endured rather than a necessary component of life's fabric to be accepted, even embraced. "Giving in" to suffering by allowing oneself the experience of deep, protracted grieving was an expression of weakness, not, as Calvinism insisted, the source of "the strength and courage to face one's condition openly and to fulfill final obligations" (231).

In Chapter 3, we quoted Thomas Reynolds's (2008) description of the core truth of personhood: "we are incomplete, vulnerable, and need others to be complete" (106). Such a description would be anathema to the Victorians, sounding as it does like a prescription for weakness and failure. But weakness and strength are not an either/or choice. They are inextricably interwoven into each person's life by the common thread of unavoidable suffering. Stanley Hauerwas's observation (1986) also bears repeating: "Suffering is built into our condition because it is literally true that we exist only to the extent that we sustain, or 'suffer,' the existence of others" (169). Human life is lived within the tension between polarities—weakness and strength, flesh and spirit, autonomy and dependence— which cannot be fully resolved. We are, as poet and songwriter Leonard Cohen expressed it, a "tangle of matter and ghost,"[9] and likewise a tangle of weakness and strength.

The legacy of the Victorians informs our culture's preoccupation with achievement and success and the attendant categorization of persons as either winners or losers. Junior-high labels dividing the in crowd from the out crowd persist in the fear of associating with losers lest we be classified as losers ourselves. The stigma assigned to weakness and failure treats these universal human experiences as potentially infectious. We are encouraged to distance ourselves from "losers" and "the weak" because the only way for us to win is for someone else to lose, and our perceived strength can be measured only over and against someone else's weakness.

In our culture, aging itself is frequently presented as a form of failure to be resisted and, when possible, overcome. As hair turns gray or begins to thin, as skin wrinkles and folds in new ways, as vision decreases or hearing becomes more challenging, as bruises heal more slowly, joints ache, or memory becomes less "sticky," we are encouraged to purchase products and services—ranging from skin creams and other nostrums to various forms of surgery—that promise to "reverse" aging, or at least the appearance of it. In other eras these manifestations of aging were viewed as badges of honor to be embraced—"the glory of youth is their strength, but the beauty of the aged is their grey hair" (Prov. 20:29)—but in our own time, they have become a shameful concession to failure and decay. The old are weak; the old are vulnerable; the old are no longer productive or interesting.

To share in friendship or participate in community with those who have been labeled weak, frail, or unsuccessful, we must confront our fears and anxieties and make peace with these dimensions of our own being. We will all be there one day, and we need friendships with those who are preceding us in this journey to learn how to enter this stage of life with wisdom and courage. We need the gifts formed by what the culture counts as weakness to find in ourselves new forms of strength.

As long as we accept a reductionist view of older persons (particularly those journeying into dementia) centered in failure we will not be receptive to the gifts they have to offer and which we need. Stanley Hauerwas and Laura Yordy (2003) lament the manner in which we excuse the aged from obligations and expectations and the price we pay in lost wisdom:

> That the elderly are freed from such obligations in our society correlates with the view that human development ends in early adulthood, or at least in middle age. Many dominant images in American culture portray old people as set in their ways, that is, as not capable of learning anything significant, much less growing in virtue. The elderly are thus thought capable of engaging in superficial friendships with other old people through time-filling "activities" rather than in profound friendships of character. Old people are portrayed as simpler people than young adults; an old person typically is either "sweet" or "irascible," neither of which indicates the interesting and complicated character of close friends. It is as though there is little reason to get to know old people because they are not very compelling as persons. Yet what could be more important than friendship between the old and the not so old, for otherwise how will the young every know how to grow old and die? (173–74)

We return to Cole's observation that being refined by experiences of suffering and loss over time confers on the aged "the strength and courage to face one's condition openly and to fulfill final obligations" (1992, 231). Among those obligations is to confer on young friends—not just through words but also through their presence—the gift of learning how to grow old and die well.

We have repeatedly referred to religious congregations as a primary setting in which genuine intergenerational friendships, including friendships incorporating persons traveling the dementia road, may be formed and sustained. They are unique settings because they are by definition centered in things of ultimate meaning. They are settings in which questions of ethics and morality are addressed and community formation is treated with intentionality. Nevertheless, we are well aware of the challenges religious congregations face in an era in which membership and participation are declining significantly, particularly among younger adults.[10] We are also acutely aware that religious leaders often lack specific training in the needs and gifts of aging persons and that many congregations lack programs focused on older adults. Those congregations that choose to prioritize programs designed to foster abiding friendships between persons from different age cohorts and seek creative ways to fully incorporate persons journeying into early and even midstage dementia will experience a renewal of purpose, vitality, and joy that will serve as both challenge and model to wider society. We also challenge those who choose not to share in the life of a religious congregation to be intentional about building new forms of community centered in hospitality and friendship, communities that purposefully include those whom society too often regards as having little of value to offer.

My Friend and I Are Living with Dementia

> The person I am with has Alzheimer's.
>
> Please be patient.
>
> Thank you.

These simple words, accompanied by a bright illustration of a sunflower, are printed on a business-sized card available through the Alzheimer's Store (www .alzstore.com). A person shopping or dining with a friend who has dementia can discreetly display the card to those serving or assisting them, hopefully eliciting a response of patience and kindness.

Absent such a cue, the person assisting will likely struggle with confusion ("What is wrong with this woman?"), impatience ("Make up your mind; other people are waiting!"), or fear ("Is this a crazy man who might begin shouting, or even assault me?"). The card offers reassurance that the friend is "normal" even though living with some limitations, and that the interaction can be manageable, even pleasant, if accompanied by an extra measure of consideration. Given the opportunity, most persons will seek to be kind and helpful. Those who work in the service industry have become accustomed to interacting with persons living with various disabilities and special needs (persons confined to wheelchairs, persons who have Down syndrome, etc.). We argued in earlier chapters that discomfort with dementia grows in part from the fear and anxiety born of our own vulnerability. But because persons who have dementia are often removed from the normal web of human relationships, it is also true that discomfort is a product of lack of familiarity. As interactions between persons who have and do not have dementia become more common, the more at ease everyone will be with such interactions.

Anne Basting (2009) argues for the formation of a "dementia rights" movement, similar to the efforts of disability advocacy organizations that led to the Americans with Disabilities Act (ADA) of 1990. With tongue only slightly in cheek, Basting proposes distributing T-shirts with the logo *Demented!* to persons who have dementia, to reclaim a word currently used to marginalize by setting it in a bold "here I am—deal with it!" context.

With or without the assistance of T-shirts, one of the tasks of those who seek to be genuine friends to persons who have dementia is to resist the stigmatization and marginalization that removes persons who are traveling the dementia road from the social mainstream. As persons overcome their own fear in order to love their friend who is living with dementia, they become equipped to teach others to move beyond the fear and awkwardness that too often inhibit the ability to interact comfortably and positively with people whose memories have lost their "stickiness" and who often feel lost and confused. Even as most persons can now see past a wheelchair to the person who sits in it, it is possible to see past the expressions of dementia to the person within.

> Al had been a member of his Rotary club for many years. He was a larger-than-life figure—an extrovert with a hearty laugh, strong opinions, and a bawdy sense of humor who rarely missed a meeting. When he failed to attend for several months, rumors spread that his health was failing and that he had recently been diagnosed with Alzheimer's disease. When Al finally appeared for a meeting after his long absence, his friends were initially shocked to see how thin and weak he looked, but in many ways he seemed to be the same irascible character he had always been. When time came for the day's announcements, he approached the podium. "Some of you have probably heard that I have Alzheimer's disease," he said to the hushed room. "Well, I do. For a while I was too embarrassed to come to meetings. But a friend said to me that if the Rotary club could put up with me the way I was before I had Alzheimer's, they can put up with me now. I may mess some things up. I may not remember your name. But if I can deal with Alzheimer's, you bastards can, too!" He received a lengthy round of applause as he returned

to his seat. Fellow members were quick to offer to drive him to meetings. Other members offered to go through the buffet line on his behalf, and Al took special delight in complaining about the food items they had selected for him. People were careful to include him in conversations. Bit by bit, Al's dementia became simply a part of who he was rather than something to speak of in whispers. He was able to attend on an occasional basis for nearly two years before his condition worsened.

Al's story stands in dramatic contrast to the one told in our introductory chapter about the woman who demanded that she be moved to a different bowling team, with "normal" people. Which story will describe the future for persons journeying into dementia—the story written by anxiety and fear or the story written by love?

In all likelihood, dementia will become part of the shared experience of many friendships as we move toward a time in the not too distant future when 20 percent of the U.S. population will be 65 or older. We need to find creative ways to nourish and sustain friendship even as memory loss and confusion mount. This can happen only if we reject our culture's view of dementia as an individual tragedy and commit ourselves to supporting one another in this new world of aging. To do this, we must accept that we are all vulnerable creatures gifted with the opportunity to build flourishing communities where everyone can live with meaning, joy, laughter, obligation, and fulfillment.

As we wrote this book, we imagined people talking about it with their friends, either in formal groups, such as classes or book clubs, or in informal conversations, as in "I read a book and it got me thinking about . . ." We offer these questions as a way of launching conversations about the joys and challenges of aging together. Persons of all ages can join these conversations. Teens and young adults may not think of themselves as aging, but many of them know people who are living with memory loss. Also, some have begun to consider who among their friends will remain in their "social convoys" as they graduate from high school or college, and they have undoubtedly experienced tests of friendship. For those of us who are older, changes in our social convoys, tests of friendship, and awareness of friends experiencing memory loss are already present realities.

CHAPTER 1: Dilemmas of Dementia Diagnoses

1. Where do people usually find information about dementia? How accurate is it? How easily available? What can communities do to make helpful, accurate information more available?
2. Do you agree with Whitehouse and Moody (2006) when they speak of a "hardening of the categories" of diagnoses and labels for forgetfulness in later life? Do you see this happening in other realms of human experience (e.g., politics)?
3. How meaningful or important is it to distinguish among different forms of dementia? What are the risks, and the benefits, of the proliferation of diagnostic labels?

CHAPTER 2: Receiving the Diagnosis

1. What are the stories you have heard or experienced of people receiving the diagnosis of cognitive impairment or dementia?
2. How does medical culture need to change so that people receiving the diagnosis of cognitive impairment or dementia do not have to experience bewilderment and fear?
3. Is it possible to receive information about a condition for which there is no cure in a manner that inspires hope?

CHAPTER 3: Personhood

1. What informs your understanding of what defines you as a self?
2. Describe situations in which you have observed or experienced social malignancy.
3. What conditions other than dementia elicit social responses that produce excess disability?
4. In what ways have people in our time accepted the cult of normalcy? Have religious organizations mounted an adequate challenge to it?

CHAPTER 4: What Is Friendship?

1. How many people (other than family) would you be willing to turn to in times of dire need?
2. What changes have you experienced in your social convoy as you have grown older?
3. Has it become more difficult in our time to experience what Aristotle described as a complete, or virtuous, friendship? If so, what forces or situations in our culture have made this more difficult?

CHAPTER 5: When Our Friends Travel the Dementia Road

1. Is there someone in your life who is traveling the dementia road? What are the greatest challenges (including those within yourself) you have experienced in your effort to maintain what Aristotle called a complete, or virtuous, friendship?
2. What puts you in your "joy zone"? Do you have at least one friend who knows you well enough to help you experience your joy zone if you take the journey into dementia? What steps do you need to take to identify your joy zone and share it with others?
3. How are friendships tested as we grow older? What resources are available to help our friendships withstand the tests of time?

CHAPTER 6: Dementia Fear and Anxiety

1. Why is cognitive decline so much more frightening and anxiety-provoking than physical decline?
2. How have you observed dementia fearmongering in your everyday life (e.g., fundraising, advertising, the popular media)? If so, how were you affected?
3. Have you ever inadvertently contributed to the stigma associated with cognitive decline?

CHAPTER 7: Beyond Fear and Anxiety

1. In what ways have you observed persons who have dementia continuing to exercise agency as they act to meet certain goals? How have they shown you that they are agents in their relationships with others?

2. Have you ever observed how the two models of fear for the self can limit people's ability to love? Recall that one describes people who have trouble trusting others, so they put great effort into maintaining boundaries in relationships. The other describes insecure people who do not trust themselves and yield to others' control.

3. How can we realistically acknowledge the two models of fear for the self and yet be guided by love and compassion in our relationships?

CHAPTER 8: The Flourishing Community

1. Has *obligation* taken on a negative meaning in our time? If so, is it worth reclaiming as essential for friendship and community life?

2. Has your experience of community been enriched by the inclusion of persons typically regarded as being different in some way? What has been your experience of ostracism of persons the community finds threatening or disturbing?

3. In our time, we have a hospitality industry, and yet the actual practice of hospitality can be challenging. What are the risks and rewards of authentic hospitality?

CHAPTER 9: Congregations as Schools for Friendship

1. If you are discussing this chapter in a congregational setting, discuss how your congregation teaches people about the meaning and practice of friendship. Does this include persons who have dementia?

2. In what sense is it legitimate to talk about faithful, committed friendship as subversive in the context of the culture in which we live today?

3. How can congregations provide spiritual accompaniment to persons who are living with dementia?

4. If a congregation committed to directing more resources to the spiritual needs and gifts of persons in midlife and beyond, what would you see as the highest priorities for use of these resources?

CHAPTER 10: The Things That Abide

1. Have you had the experience of being treated as an "it" rather than a "Thou?" Have you ever treated someone else as an "it" rather than a "Thou?" Have you ever been guilty of perceiving a friend with dementia as an "it?"

2. How can Miroslav Volf's image of the "drama of embrace" guide us in forming and maintaining friendships with people experiencing memory loss?

3. Is there a difference between having faith in your friend and being faithful to your friend? How is each expressed?

4. What are the "focal things" that you have practiced in your life (for better or for worse) that will endure as a part of your selfhood as you grow older?

CHAPTER 11: Practicing Friendship in the "Thin Places"

1. What have been your experiences of being in or meeting others in the "thin places" of life?
2. Review Aristotle's five components of virtuous, or complete, friendship and discuss how a friend's memory loss challenges us to maintain these components of friendship.
3. Within your local community, how can people encourage conversation and other forms of communication with persons who have memory loss? Within your local community, how can ties with persons living with dementia be strengthened?

CHAPTER 12: Memory, Forgetting, and the Present Time

1. How can we learn to live in the moment with our friend who no longer remembers the story of our friendship?
2. Thinking about the story of the poker group, have you already experienced the challenge of needing to reconfigure gatherings with your aging friends? What are some creative strategies for reconfiguring gatherings that include friends who have memory loss?
3. How can we find the courage to move through anxiety and fear to love?
4. What changes in local institutions and the wider society are necessary for us to treat dementia as part of our shared experience of aging together rather than as a private family matter?

INTRODUCTION

1. Much controversy centers on the language used to describe progressive forgetfulness. We employ the common term *dementia,* but we recognize that some scholars believe it to be pejorative, especially when persons are described as *demented.* Margaret Morganroth Gullette (2010) suggested that there is so much terror about dementia running through our culture that the very word is starting to sound like hate speech to her.

2. For a comprehensive history of popular and medical views on dementia, including the shift in the 1960s to the specific diagnosis of Alzheimer's disease, see Ballenger 2006.

3. This condition is beginning to be called "young-onset Alzheimer's disease" instead of "early-onset Alzheimer's disease" to reduce confusion with persons in their sixties, seventies, or eighties who are in the "early stage" of Alzheimer's disease.

4. This information comes from the Websites of the National Institutes on Aging, the Alzheimer's Association, and Alzheimer's Disease International, which is located in Great Britain. Prevalence numbers for diseases can vary according to how they are obtained and for what purposes (e.g., an organization trying to raise money for combating a disease might emphasize the higher estimates). As a comparison to the numbers cited for dementia and Alzheimer's disease, the Centers for Disease Control and Prevention stated that in 2003, more than 1 million people in the United States are living with HIV/AIDS, and in 2007 the Joint United Nations Programme on HIV/AIDS estimated that 33 million persons worldwide have HIV/AIDS.

5. See, e.g., the Website of the National Institute on Aging (www.nia.nih.gov). In a section called "the changing brain in AD," a graphic portrayal of loss and decline illustrates the diverging pathways of healthy aging and what can only be presumed from this drawing to be unhealthy aging. Curiously, the line for healthy aging (which shows a slight trend downward around age 80) ends before the label "death," unlike the one indicating Alzheimer's disease, which stops at death.

6. Robert Putnam's *Bowling Alone* (2006) first appeared as a journal article and later as a book that prompted widespread discussion in the popular media. Putnam, a sociologist, argued that his data showed how the bonds of community have frayed as voluntary

organizations attract fewer participants and people have less time to be involved in traditional group-based leisure pursuits like bowling leagues. Of course, this was not a new argument, but the image of people going to bowling alleys by themselves (regardless of how often this actually occurs) struck a chord.

7. Peter Whitehouse lists several conditions that can cause forgetfulness in older persons: depression, hypothyroidism, epilepsy (and the drugs used to control it), calcium deficiency, and alcoholism. He also includes a very helpful chapter on preparing for a doctor's visit for persons concerned about memory problems. Whitehouse believes that what we commonly call Alzheimer's disease is not a distinct disease; rather, normal brain aging has been "medicalized." He argues that we need to change our attitudes and the stories we tell about aging and forgetfulness. See Whitehouse and George 2008.

8. Linda Clare and colleagues at Bangor University in Wales do research in which they collaborate with people living with early-stage dementia instead of assigning them a number and treating them as if they were interchangeable. In other words, this research preserves personhood. In one study, Clare and colleagues inquired about the experiences of identity among people with early-stage dementia who participate in an online community called the Dementia Advocacy and Support International (DASNI). A DASNI member used the term *dementia land* to describe the new territory entered upon diagnosis and the attendant feelings of frustration, loss, loneliness, isolation, and uncertainty. See Clare, Rowlands, and Quin 2008.

9. This metaphor of the land of the well comes from Susan Sontag, who famously wrote, "Everyone who is born holds dual citizenship, in the kingdom of the well and in the kingdom of the sick. Although we all prefer to use only the good passport, sooner or later each of us is obliged, at least for a spell, to identify ourselves as citizens of that other place" (1977, 3).

10. Kenneth Gergen is one of the best-known psychologists writing about postmodernism; see Gergen 2001. In gerontology, Ruth E. Ray's excellent essay (1996) succinctly presents postmodern thinking. Postmodernism is usually debated in the ivory towers of academia and sometimes lacks obvious connections to the ways ordinary people live. Robert Kastenbaum (1993) disabuses us of that notion in an application of critical theory to a case study of the role of older adults in resisting the establishment in Arizona of a paid holiday in honor of Martin Luther King Jr.

11. Communitarianism, an idea once discussed only in the lofty reaches of academia, became fodder for cultural critics in the popular media in the 1990s as President Clinton took up the call for a strengthening of social capital. Sometimes portrayed as an expression of liberalism (e.g., when it was used to support arguments for the need for investment in environmental protection and public education) and at other times as being a fancy edifice for conservative arguments for "values education" and "faith-based" social programs, communitarianism now seems to have receded behind the ivy-covered walls of academia and social policy think tanks. We have no wish to reignite the "either/or" battles of the late twentieth / early twenty-first century, but neither do we want to ignore the challenges to and opportunities for meaningful community life posed by the demographics of age.

12. For one of the best-known critiques of American individualism as shaped by psychology (especially the anthropology espoused in Freud's psychoanalytic theory), see Philip Rieff 1966.

13. Ernest Becker (1973) argues that death infuses human consciousness, but to maintain self-esteem and support the structures of worldviews, human beings flee from the terror of death. Becker's classic work forms the foundation for social scientific research testing terror management theory. As we explain in our chapter on dementia anxiety, there are close psychological connections between the terror of death and the terror of dementia.

CHAPTER 1 · Dilemmas of Dementia Diagnoses

1. The National Institute on Aging sponsors the Alzheimer's Disease Education and Referral Center Website, which contains information about publications that can be downloaded: www.nia.nih.gov/Alzheimers/. This site contains much biomedical information, and it frames Alzheimer's disease as a growing national problem defined in terms of financial burdens on governments and emotional burdens on families. The Alzheimer's Association Website provides useful information about the diagnosis and treatment of Alzheimer's disease: www.alz.org. The Website of the National Institute of Neurological Disorders and Stroke (www.ninds.nih.gov/index.htm) can be easily searched for information about Lewy body disease, frontotemporal dementia, Parkinson's dementia, and vascular dementia. Be warned, however, that all the Websites for these diagnostic categories include phrases like "there is no cure" and "the outcome is poor."

2. Many important writings in the medical humanities have made the distinction between disease and illness. Two of the early important works are by Kleinman 1988 and Frank 1991.

3. One important source of the information included in this section on "kinds of dementia" is the chapter by Welsh-Bohmer and Warren in *Geriatric Neuropsychology* 2006. The chapter by Cato and Crosson provided information about Parkinson's disease dementia and vascular dementia, and Smith and Rush contributed a chapter on normal aging and mild cognitive impairment.

4. Some scholars and scientists believe that young-onset Alzheimer's disease, which can emerge in the third or fourth decades of life, may one day be viewed as completely different from the Alzheimer's disease that typically expresses itself in the seventh or eighth decades of life. Peter Whitehouse and Daniel George (2008) present a case for this position.

5. For a collection of articles on the history of the concept of Alzheimer's disease, including two that describe cases Dr. Alzheimer studied, see Whitehouse, Maurer, and Ballenger 2000.

6. There are many excellent sources of information about the neuropathology of Alzheimer's disease and other dementias. Increasingly, articles on this subject appear in popular media outlets, including online news stories. Epidemiologist David Snowdon (2001) explains brain changes and dementia within the context of a fascinating, humane

tale of science and spirituality. *Aging with Grace* is the story of the "nun study," in which elderly members of the School Sisters of Notre Dame volunteered for frequent cognitive and physical tests and agreed to allow their brains to be autopsied. Findings from these remarkable women continue to confound dementia researchers, for some who showed considerable accumulation of plaques, tangles, and neuronal death continued to function with few signs of dementia, while others with less neuropathology had many such signs.

7. Research on MCI has been accumulating rapidly since the dawn of the twenty-first century. The person most commonly recognized as bringing MCI to the attention of clinicians and researchers is Dr. Ronald Petersen, of the Mayo Clinic. He offered early clinical descriptions of how MCI is experienced, and he asserts that his research indicates it to be an early form of Alzheimer's disease. See, e.g., Petersen 2004.

8. Researchers at the Center for Gerontology at Virginia Tech have produced an excellent, accessible brochure for families and friends of people experiencing memory difficulties that might be classified as MCI: www.gerontology.vt.edu/docs/Gerontology_MCI_final.pdf.

9. The entire issue of *Philosophy, Psychiatry, and Psychology* 13 (1) (2006) was devoted to the controversy over mild cognitive impairment. As the editor of the issue, Julian Hughes, put it, contemporary arguments about MCI reflect the old struggle between the natural sciences and the human sciences. MCI may become a category of medical diagnosis, but it is also a label that changes the ways we view people who have the diagnosis, and it is a label that reveals how our culture responds to aging. Is the most important characteristic of the aging human being defined by the change in how much and how quickly we remember? Many people would say no.

CHAPTER 2 · Receiving the Diagnosis

1. These legal protections were enacted in 1996 as the Health Insurance Portability and Accountability Act, better known as HIPAA. They guard the security and privacy of medical information. LGBT (lesbian/gay/bisexual/transgendered) persons who live in states that do not recognize the legality of their relationship have to endure many hurdles in order to accompany their partners in medical environments. Persons who have lived "out of the closet" for many years sometimes have to retreat to secrecy when they relocate to assisted-living or skilled-nursing residences. A comparison of the Websites of the Alzheimer's Association in the United States (www.alz.org) and the Alzheimer's Society of United Kingdom (http://alzheimers.org.uk) shows the lag in U.S. responses to the LGBT community that is dealing with dementia. The search engine for the Alzheimer's Society produces a number of "hits" when "gays/lesbians" is entered; the search engine for the Alzheimer's Association produces nothing with the same search. The Alzheimer's Society has a dedicated page for the LGBT community (http://alzheimers.org.uk/gaycarers) with information about support groups, help lines, legal issues, and residential care.

2. For an excellent theoretical and empirical account of how religious coping can be both adaptive and maladaptive, see Pargament 1997.

3. Several Websites claim to offer personal genetic testing for a number of diseases and what one site calls "health traits." Usually people submit a sample of spit, and the

analysis appears several weeks later on a supposedly secure Website. This process is called "personal genome service" and appears to be marketed to tech-savvy young adults.

4. Perhaps this is not so odd after all, given that researchers are now searching for various biomarkers of dementia that appear in the blood, urine, cerebrospinal fluid, brain images, and genes of young and middle-aged adults long before any symptoms emerge.

CHAPTER 3 · Personhood

1. This group eventually became the Pioneer Network. See www.pioneernetwork.net.

2. Robert Kastenbaum (2004) described a similar problem among those who work with people who are dying. He called it "status contamination."

3. This film can be ordered from www.almosthomeoutreach.org.

4. See Deborah Blum's book *Love at Goon Park* (2002) for a detailed, lively discussion of Harlow's life and research. "Goon Park" is what students and faculty called the psychology building at the University of Wisconsin in Madison because its address was 600 N. Park.

5. For a book that engagingly describes studies of relationships from the perspectives of developmental, psychoanalytic, social, and neurological psychology, see Lewis, Amini, and Lannon 2000.

6. Namaste Care (from the Sanskrit word that means a respectful greeting) has been developed as a way of offering meaningful activities to persons with advanced dementia. It can include soft music, dimmed lights, loving touch, pleasant fragrances, and other forms of relaxing but attentive stimulation offered by caregivers. It has been shown to have positive benefits in terms of decreased agitation and increased social interaction. See Simard and Volicer 2010.

7. Other terms used to describe this situation are *Pygmalian effect, self-fulfilling prophecy,* and *stereotype threat.* Each of these phrases refers to the fact that people often behave in ways that reflect others' expectations of them. We find it fascinating that so many different terms have been applied to the same phenomenon, which is, perhaps, an indication of its pervasiveness and power. For a review of research on the effects of this behavior on persons with Alzheimer's disease, see Scholl and Sabat 2008.

8. What should we call the person who takes on primary responsibility for caring for a person who has dementia? Most of the time, we refer to this individual as a *caregiver.* Caregivers are described as being either family members (usually a spouse, daughter, or son) or persons who are paid to give care. Although we refer to *paid caregivers* in this book, we are increasingly sensitive to the one-sidedness of the term *caregiver.* Caring implies a relationship, and that is why we prefer the phrase *care partnering.* There is another reason for bringing this term into the way we talk about care. Not all persons who give care to loved ones in their homes are family members. Although gay and lesbian persons caring for their partners have received little notice in the literature on dementia care, as we noted in Chapter 2 (n. 1), some organizations are beginning to offer them support, most notably the Alzheimer's Society of Great Britain.

9. Today many articles, book chapters, and books are available about spirituality and dementia. See, e.g., McCurdy 1998 and Allen and Coleman 2006.

10. In addition to the works by Reinders (2008), Reynolds (2008), and Swinton (2004) cited in the following sections, see also Swinton and Brock 2007.

11. A common definition of faith is "remembering God and being mindful of God in all that we do." Hauerwas suggests that such an inadequate definition leads persons to fear that they will not be able to sustain a faith when memory fails.

12. A version of Hauerwas's remarks can be found in the documentary film *There Is a Bridge* (Chicago: Memory Bridge, 2007). The version offered here comes from personal conversation.

13. John Swinton edited a collection of essays that represents a dialogue with Hauerwas on his theology of disability; the collection includes a number of responses written by Hauerwas to others' reflections on his work. See Swinton 2004.

14. *Hamlet,* act 2, scene 2, lines 303–5.

15. *De Generis ad Litteram* 6.12.

16. *Summa Theologia,* 1a, q-95, a.6.

17. Luther, *Works,* 1. 61.

18. E.g., Exodus 9:14–16; Leviticus 21:17–24; Matthew 3:7–12.

19. See Mark 10:52; Luke 17:19.

20. See Psalm 73:2–5; Job 42:7–8; Matthew 5:45.

21. See Isaiah 29:18–19; Luke 14:15–24.

22. Reynolds borrows his version of this term from Hauerwas (1986), who expressed it as "The Tyranny of Normality."

CHAPTER 4 · What Is Friendship?

1. Gerontologist H. R. (Rick) Moody sometimes refers to "well elders" in this group as the "well-derly."

2. An alphabetical and admittedly random list that might be generated by looking at the undergraduate majors of today's well-known gerontologists would include art, biology, computer science, economics, history, geography, literature, kinesiology, music, philosophy, political science, psychology, sociology, theater, and women's studies. Graduate degrees can range from advanced work in these and other fields, to professional training in medicine, nursing, pharmacy, occupational and physical therapy, and social work.

3. This idea of "standing grounds" can be stretched to include many of the defining characteristics of persons in our postmodern era. For example, although the vast majority of gerontologists are from white, European heritages, recent years have found more persons representing various racial and ethnic groups coming into the field. Gerontologists vary in gender, sexual orientation, class background (if not so dramatically in current class identification), and of course, age. Thus, it is important to recognize when talking about their standing grounds that the Ph.D. in her thirties may have a different view of aging and how to study it than the researcher nearing retirement with a long history of researching and writing about later life.

4. A widely used organizational framework for research on adult friendships can be found in Adams and Blieszner 1994.

5. It might interest some readers to know that Rebecca Adams is a well-known expert on "Deadheads," people who formed lasting friendships and an enduring community based upon their love of the band, the Grateful Dead. See, e.g., Adams and Sardiello 2000.

6. The literature produced by this controversy over "activity theory" versus "disengagement theory" is vast. Disengagement theory was launched in Cumming and Henry 1961. It is more difficult to cite one particular work that presented the activity argument, but one example is Rosow 1967.

7. See McFadden and Atchley (2001), in which the editors asked a group of gerontologists representing many disciplines to reflect on the meaning of time.

8. There are many translations of the *Nicomachean Ethics,* and this work can also be found in various forms online (see, e.g., http://classics.mit.edu/Aristotle/nicomachean .html). We are using the English translation by H. Rackham (1975).

9. This quote comes from Nouwen's book, *Bread for the Journey* (1997). This is a "daybook of wisdom and faith" and so has no page numbers. This selection is intended to be read on January 7.

10. Adams and colleagues also noted gender differences in researchers who study older adults' friendship. Female researchers are more likely to employ what Adams et al. describe as "communal" methodologies with open-ended survey questions, to focus on friendship dyads or networks, and to pay attention to multiple characteristics of friendship. In contrast, male researchers use "agentic" approaches, which force participants to answer according to a set pattern (1 if you strongly disagree, 5 if you strongly agree) and do not focus on multiple friendship types. These authors do not take an "essentialist" position on this finding, meaning they do not think that there is something about gender that causes people to use one approach or the other. Rather, they suggest that men may have better access to resources to conduct large-scale survey research. See Adams et al. 2006.

CHAPTER 5 · When Our Friends Travel the Dementia Road

1. In addition to Matthews 1986 and Rook 1989, see also Blieszner and Adams 1998. Their interviews with people age 55–84 showed that despite a number of identified difficulties, older people are reluctant to terminate friendships. Another work that relied on interviews to examine late-life-friendship predicaments is Rawlins 1994.

2. See, e.g., Albert, Cohen, and Koff 1991 and Zandi, Cooper, and Garrison 1992.

3. One chapter in Basting (2009) reviews recent autobiographies written by people who have dementia. The courageous people who have recorded their personal narratives of dementia are inspiring activists to campaign for radical changes in how our culture views persons who have the dementia diagnosis.

CHAPTER 6 · Dementia Fear and Anxiety

1. A follow-up study in 2010 found the fear has not abated. Google "What America Thinks: MetLife Foundation Alzheimer's Survey" to find the report.

2. This survey was done in conjunction with a series of four documentary films made for HBO on the subject of Alzheimer's disease. See www.hbo.com/alzheimers/downloads/Census.pdf. The films can be found at www.hbo.com/alzheimers/the-films.html, along with fifteen supplemental videos on specific topics related to primarily to dementia research.

3. Psychologists use the word *valence* to refer to the direction an emotion takes, that is, whether it is experienced as positive or as negative.

4. Many of the so-called difficult behaviors of persons who have dementia—such as striking others or shouting—can best be understood as expressions of emotion arising from the perception of threat in the environment. These behaviors often occur when the person is feeling most vulnerable and least able to escape threat, as, for example, when being bathed. Understanding emotion as resulting from an interaction between a person and some situation in the environment helps us get beyond seeing these difficult behaviors as resulting solely from whatever is happening in the brain as a result of dementia. As we note later in the chapter, these behaviors also arise when people feel that they are being treated as if they are already dead.

5. It will be interesting to observe the public's reactions in coming years as information about research showing the start of brain aging in young adulthood becomes more widely known. One authority has written that "cognitive declines begin by the 20s and 30s in healthy highly educated adults and continue into later ages independent of known pathology" (Finch 2009, 515). The vital intellectual engagement of so many older people is testimony to the brain's reserve capacity and plasticity, both of which are supported by genetics, good diet, exercise, cognitive and social stimulation, and control of vascular problems like hypertension and high cholesterol. Finch also adds that air pollution is being implicated in accelerated brain aging.

6. For a comprehensive treatment of research testing terror management theory, see Greenberg, Koole, and Pyszczynski 2004. Because this is an endnote, Susan will add the personal comment that she never imagined she would see *experimental* and *existential psychology* in the same book title.

7. Melissa Lunsman O'Connor; see Lunsman 2006.

8. Many forces combined to create public concern about Alzheimer's disease. Together, they are sometimes labeled the "Alzheimer's disease movement." For two excellent histories of this phenomenon, see Fox 1989 and Beard 2004.

CHAPTER 7 · Beyond Fear and Anxiety

1. Another recommendation for our imaginary friend (or the real readers of this book) is Ballenger et al. 2009. The answer to the question, "Do we have a pill for it?" is yes and no. Yes, there are many pills prescribed for dementia, but, as Peter Rabins suggests in the last chapter, we have only "modest treatments" (253). He is referring to pharmacological interventions that have the goal either of improving cognitive performance on various tests or of preventing further cognitive decline, again as measured by specific tests. On the other hand, we do know a lot about nurturing overall life quality for persons who have dementia and those who care for them. That is the focus of Basting 2009.

2. Christine Bryden (2005) described her experience of dementia using the metaphor of dance to describe her sense of being a partner with her husband, Paul, as she struggled with the symptoms of dementia and her depression about the diagnosis. Later, after the book had been out for several years, she told of becoming a less active partner: "more scrambled, more anxious, more distressed; less able to express my needs, less able to communicate what I am feeling" (Bryden and MacKinlay 2008, 139).

3. The Gifford lectures rotate among the Universities of Edinburgh, Glasgow, Aberdeen, and St. Andrews. One of the authors of this book (John) had the honor of attending the Gifford lectures delivered by Stanley Hauerwas at the University of St. Andrews in 2001.

4. This description, given by social scientists to categorize people, does not reflect the actuality of interdependence for which we are making the case here.

5. "Activities of daily living," or ADLs, in the lingo of professional care partners and researchers, include the things people normally do in the course of a day, such as brushing teeth, bathing, going to the toilet, getting up from a chair and moving about, getting dressed, and eating.

6. The description of Marge in the kitchen is an example of Stephen Sabat's claim that persons who have Alzheimer's disease are "semiotic subjects." By this he means that they are "individuals who can act intentionally given their interpretations of the circumstances in which they find themselves; they are people who can evaluate their own behavior and the behavior of others in accordance with socially agreed-upon standards of propriety and reason (2001, 171).

7. In case any readers are wondering how this book can have anything to do with religion (as dictated by the terms of the Gifford endowment), we point them to Macmurray's position in *Persons in Relation* that "religion cannot be understood from the standpoint of the isolated agent, but only when we are considering persons in relation" (151). This is a book about the philosophy of religion—about religion as a human activity—and not about any particular expression of religion. Macmurray compares "illusory religion," which promotes defensive egocentricity and fear of life, to "real religion," which, "so far as it is concerned with oneself, it is for the sake of the other" (171).

8. In a sociopolitical sense, de Rivera argues that the first type of manifestation of fear for the self leads to the aggressive individualism of some cultures, whereas the second type is present in collectivist cultures. Both are caricatures, of course, for in both types of culture, one finds persons who exemplify the third model of the self, in which concern for the other dominates fear for the self.

9. Fear of dementia in Western, individualistic cultures focuses on the loss of autonomy. In Eastern, collectivist cultures, the fear focuses on the loss of an honored place within the community. We realize that this distinction between individualist and collectivist cultures is overly broad and is hotly debated by scholars. However, we have known Hmong families (persons who fled Laos at the end of the Vietnam War, many of whom now live in the upper Midwest) who describe the shame they feel when an elder has memory loss and thus can no longer function as a vital member of the community. Hmong elders are expected to provide moral leadership; the inability to do this by virtue of progressive forgetfulness excludes them from their role within the clan. One granddaughter of a man who was living with dementia described how her grandmother drew

the shades of their house and, with her husband, became reclusive, because of the shame of not being able to fulfill social expectations. For a Japanese perspective on memory loss written by an anthropologist, see Traphagan 2000.

CHAPTER 8 · The Flourishing Community

1. See www.slate.com/id/2380/.

2. As described by Case and Williams (2004), the word *ostracism* comes from the ancient Greek practice of voting to exile people with political ambitions who threatened the accepted order of things. Citizens would cast votes with shards of pottery called *ostraca*. In effect, exiles were voted "on the island" rather than "off the island" (as in a popular reality television show).

CHAPTER 9 · Congregations as Schools for Friendship

1. Residents of the Legacy (not its real name) typically represent a relatively high socioeconomic status. However, many of the dynamics of community they experience, such as negotiations with staff and administrators over maintaining their sense of independence, are reflected in an ethnographic study by Pia Kontos of a facility for low-income elders in Canada. See Kontos 1998.

2. One chapter of the book addresses dementia and offers suggestions for a variety of congregational programs to educate people about medical issues and community services and resources. Bennett and Hale also suggest that congregations should find ways to offer family respite care.

3. This is more descriptive of white, middle-class congregations. Most studies find higher levels of religious participation, religious coping, and spirituality among older African Americans and Caribbean blacks than among whites. See, e.g., Taylor, Chatters, and Jackson 2007.

4. See www.seniorsplace.org for more information about the history of the organization and the growth of its programs.

5. Much good work is being done in Great Britain, where many programs incorporating the perspective of the "new culture" of dementia care are being adapted by religious groups. The Christian Council on Ageing (www.ccoa/org.uk) publishes *Dementia Newsletter*, which gives information about congregational programs and reviews relevant books, news articles, and Websites.

6. For more information about Meet Me at MoMA, see www.moma.org/learn/programs/alzheimers.

CHAPTER 10 · The Things That Abide

1. Personal communication.

2. For a collection of essays that explore this theme, see McKim 1997.

3. Less progressive residential care homes treat worship as an activity and view the worship leader (usually a local clergyperson who is not trained to work with persons who

have dementia) as taking charge of an activity so that the staff can take a break. Residents are brought to the service and left there. Family and friends do not participate, and there is no sense of community before, during, or after the service.

4. A paper by Zinnbauer, Pargament, and coauthors who were Pargament's doctoral students at the time is one of our favorite efforts to differentiate and define religion and spirituality. Not only is it well argued and supported by data collected from a diverse sample, but it also has a clever, descriptive title. See Zinnbauer et al. 1997.

5. From L'Arche USA Website: http://larcheusa.org/.

6. Nouwen (1997) later wrote a book about his relationship with Adam.

CHAPTER 11 · Practicing Friendship in the "Thin Places"

1. Psychologists have studied thresholds since the late nineteenth century, particularly in terms of the line between what we can see, hear, taste, smell, and feel and the sensory experiences that lie just beyond our ability to be aware of them. These are sometimes described as *subliminal*. Interestingly, the first psychologist who developed methods for studying thresholds, the great German physiologist Gustav Fechner, was both a scientist and a mystic. He described his "day self" and his "night self" as separated by a psychological "thin place."

2. Friedell's essays about his experiences having dementia can be found on his Website: www.morrisfriedell.com.

3. Richard Taylor gives lectures all over the world encouraging persons who have dementia to "speak up and speak out" about their experiences. He posts blog entries to his Website: www.richardtaylorphd.com.

4. The "culture change" movement in long-term care has inspired a new way of seeing residents, and it supports recruitability. Facilities that have embraced culture change reject the model of care that says employees must be moved from unit to unit so they do not grow attached to residents. Residents' life stories are shared with staff; often a "memory box" outside a bedroom contains important items reflecting the identity of the person who resides there. As long as they maintain ethical boundaries, staff members are urged to allow themselves to be recruited by residents. Some residents do this more easily, but even the most "difficult" residents in these progressive facilities usually have recruited at least one staff member.

5. Most of the publications about communication with persons who have dementia focus either on family members or on paid care partners. We have found little information directed toward friends. However, there is a short document with many good, practical suggestions, available online from the Alzheimer Scotland "Action on Dementia" program: "I'll get by with a little help from my friends: Information for friends of people with dementia." It can be accessed at www.alzscot.org/pages/info/friends.htm.

6. Guides for pastors wishing to design services that meet the spiritual needs of persons who have moderate to severe dementia are beginning to appear. One of the best is Shamy 2003.

7. Jesse Ballenger noted an important difference between these individuals and others with disabilities and stigmatized identities (e.g., persons who have HIV/AIDS) in that

they "will not be able to ground their selfhood in the dominant values of our culture—independence, self-control and productivity—as have other disability activists. They must also find ways to value, or at least reconcile themselves to dependency, contingency, and loss" (2008).

8. Snyder's book is divided into three parts: listening, speaking, and responding. In the "speaking" section, Snyder (a social worker) relates what happened when she invited seven persons with memory loss to "speak their minds." Their stories, interspersed with Snyder's sensitive and insightful reflections, teach readers how to listen well and how to respond in order to create a better world for people who are living with dementia.

CHAPTER 12 · Memory, Forgetting, and the Present Time

1. Gerontologists refer to aging in place as the desire of older persons to grow old, and perhaps even die, in the same homes (or communities) in which they have lived for decades. Contrary to the image of people taking off for warmer climates as soon as they retire, most older people remain in their communities. Even those who do relocate often return once they are widowed or begin to experience physical or mental frailty.

2. There are a number of Websites devoted to NORCs, but one of the best is sponsored by the Jewish Federations of North America: www.norcs.com.

3. Micheal Winerip, "A coffee shop that is so much more," www.nytimes.com/2010/01/03/fashion/03genb.html.

4. See, e.g., www.cohousing.org.

5. See http://blog.nielsen.com/nielsenwire/nielsen-news/americans-watching-more-tv-than-ever/.

6. This is what some psychologists call *flow,* the optimal experience of engaging in an activity for its own sake and not some future reward, an activity in which one feels so involved that time feels transformed. See Csikszentmihalyi 1990.

7. Dr. Desai established a transformative practice in geriatric psychiatry in our community. Through his establishment of the Alzheimer's Center of Excellence, he was not only engaged in clinical medicine but also devoted to educating the public about possibilities for living well with memory loss. His patients, their families, and his colleagues were all saddened when he decided to return to academic medicine, although they softened their grief with the hope that he would pass his wise, holistic approach to treating persons who are living with dementia to future generations of geriatric psychiatrists. See Desai and Grossberg 2010.

8. Randy Cohen, "The public ethicist," www.nytimes.com/2009/11/29/magazine/29FOB-ethicist-t.html.

9. Leonard Cohen, "The Window" (1979).

10. See the Report on the U.S. Religious Landscape Survey, conducted by the Pew Forum on Religion and Public Life, http://religions.pewforum.org.

REFERENCES

Aartsen, M. J., T. van Tilburg, C. H. M. Smits, and K. C. P. M. Knipscheer. 2004. A longitudinal study of the impact of physical and cognitive decline on the personal network in old age. *Journal of Social and Personality Relationships* 21:249–66.

Achenbaum, W. A. 2005. *Older Americans, vital communities: A bold vision for societal aging.* Baltimore: Johns Hopkins University Press.

Adams, R. G. 1997. Friendship patterns among older women. In J. M. Coyle, ed., *Handbook on women and aging,* 400–417. Westport, CT: Greenwood Press.

Adams, R. G., J. Berggren, L. Docherty, K. Ruffin, and C. P. Wright. 2006. Gender-of-author differences in study design of older adult friendship surveys. *Personal Relationships* 13:501–20.

Adams, R. G., and R. Blieszner. 1994. An integrative conceptual framework for friendship research. *Journal of Social and Personal Relationships* 11:163–84.

Adams, R. G., R. Blieszner, and B. De Vries. 2000. Definitions of friendship in the third age: Age, gender, and study location effects. *Journal of Aging Studies* 14:117–33.

Adams, R. G., and R. Sardiello. 2000. *You ain't gonna learn what you don't know.* Walnut Creek, CA: AltaMira Press.

Ainsworth, M. D. S., M. C. Blehar, E. Waters, and S. Wall. 1978. *Patterns of attachment: A psychological study of the strange situation.* Hillsdale, NJ: Erlbaum.

Albert, M. S., C. Cohen, and E. Koff. 1991. Perception of affect in patients with dementia of the Alzheimer type. *Archives of Neurology* 48:791–95.

Allen, F. B., and P. G. Coleman. 2006. Spiritual perspectives on the person with dementia: Identify and personhood. In J. C. Hughes, S. J. Louw, and S. R. Sabat, eds., *Dementia: Mind, meaning, and the person,* 205–21. New York: Oxford University Press.

Aniskiewicz, A. S. 2007. *Psychotherapy for neuropsychological challenges.* New York: Jason Aronson.

Aristotle. 1975. *The Nicomachean ethics.* Trans. H. Rackham. Cambridge, MA: Harvard University Press.

Atchley, R. C. 1989. A continuity theory of normal aging. *Gerontologist* 29:183–90.

Atchley, R. C. 1999. *Continuity and adaptation in aging: Creating positive experiences.* Baltimore: Johns Hopkins University Press.

Atchley, R. C. 2009. *Spirituality and aging.* Baltimore: Johns Hopkins University Press.

Attix, D. K., and K. A. Welsh-Bohmer, eds. 2006. *Geriatric neuropsychology: Assessment and intervention.* New York: Guilford Press.

Bakan, D. 1966. *The duality of human existence: An essay on psychology and religion.* Chicago: Rand McNally.

Ballenger, J. 2006. *Self, senility, and Alzheimer's disease in modern America: A history.* Baltimore: Johns Hopkins University Press.

Ballenger, J. 2008. Alzheimer's patients need to be engaged citizens. *Newsday,* June 21. www.newsday.com.

Ballenger, J., P. J. Whitehouse, C. G. Lyketsos, P. V. Rabins, and J. H. T. Karlawish, eds. 2009. *Treating dementia: Do we have a pill for it?* Baltimore: Johns Hopkins University Press.

Barnes, D. E., K. E. Covinsky, R. A. Whitmer, L. H. Kuller, O. L. Lopez, and K. Yaffe. 2009. Predicting risk of dementia in older adults: The late-life dementia risk index. *Neurology* 73:173–79.

Bartholomew, K.1990. Avoidance of intimacy: An attachment perspective. *Journal of Social and Personal Relationships* 7:147–78.

Bartlett, R., and D. O'Connor. 2007. From personhood to citizenship: Broadening the lens for dementia practice and research. *Journal of Aging Studies* 21:107–18.

Bassuk, S. S., T. A. Glass, and L. F. Berkman. 1999. Social disengagement and incident cognitive decline in community-dwelling elderly persons. *Annals of Internal Medicine* 131:165–73.

Basting, A. 2009. *Forget memory: Creating better lives for people with dementia.* Baltimore: Johns Hopkins University Press.

Baumeister, R. F., and M. R. Leary. 1995. The need to belong: Desire for interpersonal attachments as a fundamental human motivation. *Psychological Bulletin* 117: 497–529.

Beard, R. 2004. Advocating voice: Organisational, historical and social milieu of the Alzheimer's disease movement. *Sociology of Health and Illness* 26:797–819.

Becker, E. 1973. *The denial of death.* New York: Free Press.

Beer, F. 1998. *Julian of Norwich: Revelations of Divine love, the motherhood of God: An excerpt.* Rochester, NY: Boydell & Brewer.

Bellah, R. N., R. Madsen, W. M. Sullivan, A. Swidler, and S. M. Tipton. 1985. *Habits of the heart: Individualism and commitment in American life.* Berkeley: University of California Press.

Bennett, D. A., J. A. Schneider, Y. Tang, S. E. Arnold, and R. S. Wilson. 2006. The effect of social networks on the relation between Alzheimer's disease pathology and level of cognitive function in old people: A longitudinal cohort study. *Lancet Neurology* 5:406–12.

Bennett, R. G., and W. D. Hale. 2009. *Building healthy communities through medical-religious partnerships.* 2nd ed. Baltimore: Johns Hopkins University Press.

Berscheid, E. 1999. The greening of relationship science. *American Psychologist* 54: 260–66.

Birren, J. E. 2001. Foreword. In Kenyon, Clark, and deVries, *Narrative gerontology,* vii–ix.

Blakney, R. B. 1941. *Meister Eckhart: A modern translation.* New York: Harper & Row.

Blieszner, R., and Adams, R. G. 1998. Problems with friends in old age. *Journal of Aging Studies* 12:223–38.

Blum, D. 2002. *Love at Goon Park.* Cambridge, MA: Perseus Publishing.

Borgmann, A. 1984. *Technology and the character of contemporary life.* Chicago: University of Chicago Press.

Bowlby, J. 1969–80. *Attachment and loss.* 3 vols. New York: Basic Books.

Brock, F. 2008. Houston faith communities collaborate on memory care day center. *Generations* 32:42–43.

Brod, M., A. L. Stewart, L. Sands, and P. Walton. 1999. Conceptualization and measurement of quality of life in dementia: The Dementia Quality of Life Instrument (DQoL). *Gerontologist* 39:25–35.

Brody, E. M., M. H. Kleban, M. P. Lawton, and H. A. Silverman. 1971. Excess disabilities of mentally impaired aged: Impact of individualized treatment. *Gerontologist* 11 (2, pt. 1):124–33.

Brown, S. L., R. M. Nesse, A. D. Vinokur, and D. M. Smith. 2003. Providing social support may be more beneficial than receiving it: Results from a prospective study of mortality. *Psychological Science* 14:320–27.

Bryden, C. 2005. *Dancing with dementia: My story of living positively with dementia.* Philadelphia: Jessica Kingsley Publishers.

Bryden, C., and E. MacKinlay. 2008. Dementia: A journey inwards to a spiritual self. In MacKinlay, *Ageing, disability, and spirituality,* 134–44.

Buber, M. 1970. *I and thou.* Trans. W. Kaufmann. New York: Charles Scribner's Sons.

Burgener, S. C., Y. Yang, R. Gilbert, and S. Marsh-Yant. 2008. The effects of a multimodal intervention on outcomes of persons with early-stage dementia. *American Journal of Alzheimer's Disease* 23:382–94.

Burnham, H., and E. Hogervorst. 2004. Recognition of facial expressions of emotion by patients with dementia of the Alzheimer type. *Dementia and Geriatric Cognitive Disorders* 18:75–79.

Butler, R. 1963. The life review: An interpretation of reminiscence in the aged. *Psychiatry* 26:65–76.

Cacioppo, J. T., D. G. Amaral, J. J. Blanchard, J. L. Cameron, C. S. Carter, D. Crews, et al. 2007. Social neuroscience: Progress and implications for mental health. *Perspectives on Psychological Science* 2:99–123.

Carpenter, B. 2009. "You have Alzheimer's disease": How to reveal a diagnosis and how to deal with the reactions. *Generations* 33:82–85.

Carstensen, L. L. 1992. Social and emotional patterns in adulthood: Support for socioemotional selectivity theory. *Psychology and Aging* 7:331–38.

Case, T. I., and K. D. Williams. 2004. Ostracism: A metaphor for death. In Greenberg, Koole, and Pyszczynski, *Handbook of experimental existential psychology,* 336–51.

Cato, M. A., and B. A. Crosson. 2006. Stable and slowly progressive dementias. In Attix and Welsh-Bohmer, *Geriatric neuropsychology,* 89–102.

Chen, Z., K. D. Williams, J. Fitness, and N. C. Newton. 2008. When hurt will not heal: Exploring the capacity to relive social and physical pain. *Psychological Science* 19: 789–95.

Christiansen, D. 1995. A Catholic perspective. In Kimble et al., *Aging, spirituality, and religion*, 403–16.

Chung, P. Y. F., C. Ellis-Hill, and P. G. Coleman. 2008. Carers perspectives on the activity patterns of people with dementia. *Dementia* 7:359–81.

Clare, L. 2003. Managing threats to self: Awareness in early stage Alzheimer's disease. *Social Science and Medicine* 57:1017–29.

Clare, L., T. Goater, and B. Woods. 2006. Illness representations in early-stage dementia: A preliminary investigation. *International Journal of Geriatric Psychiatry* 21:761–67.

Clare, L., I. Roth, and R. Pratt. 2005. Perceptions of change over time in early-stage Alzheimer's disease: Implications for understanding awareness and coping style. *Dementia* 4:487–520.

Clare, L., J. Rowlands, E. Bruce, C. Surr, and M. Downs. 2008a. "I don't do like I used to do": A grounded theory approach to conceptualizing awareness in people with moderate to severe dementia living in long-term care. *Social Science and Medicine* 66:2366–77.

Clare, L., J. Rowlands, E. Bruce, C. Surr, and M. Downs. 2008b. The experience of living with dementia in residential care: An interpretative phenomenological analysis. *Gerontologist* 48:711–20.

Clare, L., J. Rowlands, and R. Quin. 2008. Collective strength: The impact of developing a shared social identity in early-stage dementia. *Dementia* 7: 9–30.

Cole, T. R. 1992. *The journey of life: A cultural history of aging in America*. New York: Cambridge University Press.

Corner, L., and J. Bond. 2004. Being at risk of dementia: Fears and anxieties of older adults. *Journal of Aging Studies* 18:143–55.

Csikszentmihalyi, M. 1990. *Flow: The psychology of optimal experience*. San Francisco: HarperCollins.

Cumming, E., and W. E. Henry. 1961. *Growing old: The process of disengagement*. New York: Basic Books.

Darwin, C. 1872/1965. *The expression of emotion in man and animals*. Chicago: University of Chicago Press.

DeLashmutt, M. W. 2009. Delusions and dark materials: New atheism as naïve atheism and its challenge to theological education. *Expository Times* 120:586–93.

De Rivera, J. H. 1989. Love, fear, and justice: Transforming selves for the new world. *Social Justice Research* 3:387–426.

Desai, A., and G. T. Grossberg. 2010. *Psychiatric consultation in long-term care: A guide for health care professionals*. Baltimore: Johns Hopkins University Press.

Downs, M., L. Clare, and E. Anderson. 2008. Dementia as a biopsychosocial condition: Implications for practice and research. In R. Woods and L. Clare, eds., *Handbook of the Clinical Psychology of Aging*, 2nd ed., 145–59. West Sussex, UK: John Wiley & Sons.

Dychtwald, K. 1990. *The age wave: How the most important trend of our time can change your future*. New York: Bantam Books.

Eckhart, Meister. 1941. *Meister Eckhart: A modern translation*. Trans. R. B. Blakney. New York: Harper & Row.

Eisenberger, N. I., and M. D. Lieberman. 2004. Why rejection hurts: A common neural alarm system for physical and social pain. *Trends in Cognitive Sciences* 8:294–300.

Ellor, J. W. 1995. Elements of parish revitalization. In Kimble et al., *Aging, spirituality, and religion,* 270–83.

Erikson, E. H. 1950. *Childhood and society.* New York: W. W. Norton.

Erikson, E. H., J. M. Erikson, and H. Q. Kivnick. 1986. *Vital involvement in old age: The experience of old age in our time.* New York: W. W. Norton.

Ersner-Hershfield, H., J. A. Mikels, S. J. Sullivan, and L. L. Carstensen. 2008. Poignancy: Mixed emotional experience in the face of meaningful endings. *Journal of Personality and Social Psychology* 94:158–67.

Finch, C. E. 2009. The neurobiology of middle-age has arrived. *Neurobiology of Aging* 30:515–20.

Folkman, S., and R. S. Lazarus. 1980. An analysis of coping in a middle-aged community sample. *Journal of Health and Social Behavior* 48:150–70.

Fox, P. 1989. From senility to Alzheimer's disease: The rise of the Alzheimer's disease movement. *Milbank Quarterly* 67:58–102.

Frank, A. 1991. *At the will of the body: Reflections on illness.* New York: Houghton Mifflin.

Frank, L., A. Lloyd, J. A. Flynn, L. Kleinman, L. S. Matza, M. K. Margolis, et al. 2006. Impact of cognitive impairment on mild dementia patients and mild cognitive impairment patients and their informants. *International Psychogeriatrics* 18:151–62.

Fratiglioni, L., S. Paillard-Borg, and B. Winglad. 2004. An active and socially integrated lifestyle in late life might protect against dementia. *Lancet Neurology* 3:343–53.

Freud, S. 1917/1957. Mourning and melancholia. In *The standard edition of the complete psychological works of Sigmund Freud,* ed. J. Strachey et al., 14: 239–58. London: Hogarth Press.

Friedell, M., and C. Bryden. 2002. A word from two turtles. *Dementia* 1:131–33.

Friedman, D. A. 2001a. *Hitlavut Ruchanit*: Spiritual accompanying. In Friedman, *Jewish pastoral care,* ix–xxi.

Friedman, D. A. 2001b. Letting their faces shine: Accompanying aging people and their families. In Friedman, *Jewish pastoral care,* 286–316.

Friedman, D. A., ed. 2001. *Jewish pastoral care: A practical handbook from traditional and contemporary sources.* Woodstock, VT: Jewish Lights Publishing.

Friedman, D. A. 2003. An anchor amidst anomie: Ritual and aging. In Kimble and McFadden, *Aging, spirituality, and religion,* 134–44.

Friedman, D. A., ed. 2005. *Jewish pastoral care: A practical handbook from traditional and contemporary sources.* 2nd ed., rev. Woodstock, VT: Jewish Lights Publishing.

Friedman, D. A. 2008. *Jewish visions for aging.* Woodstock, VT: Jewish Lights Publishing.

George, D., and P. J. Whitehouse. 2009. The classification of Alzheimer's disease and mild cognitive impairment: Enriching therapeutic models through moral imagination. In Ballenger et al., *Treating dementia,* 5–24.

Gergen, K. 2001. Psychological science in a postmodern context. *American Psychologist* 56:803–13.

Gibson, F. 2004. *The past in the present: Using reminiscence in health and social care.* Baltimore: Health Professions Press.

Goffman, E. 1963. *Stigma: Notes on the management of spoiled identity.* New York: Simon & Schuster.

Greenberg, J., S. L. Koole, and T. Pyszczynski, eds. 2004. *Handbook of experimental existential psychology*. New York: Guilford Press.

Greenberg, J. R., and S. A. Mitchell. 1983. *Object relations in psychoanalytic theory*. Cambridge, MA: Harvard University Press.

Gullette, M. M. 2010. *What's age got to do with it?* Chicago: University of Chicago Press.

Hachinski, V. 2008. Shifts in thinking about dementia. *Journal of the American Medical Association* 300:2172–73.

Hafner, K. 2008. Exercise your brain, or else you'll . . . uh . . . *New York Times*, May 3. www.nytimes.com.

Hallahan, L. 2008. On relationships not things: Exploring disability and spirituality. In MacKinlay, *Ageing, disability, and spirituality*, 94–105.

Harris, P. B., ed. 2002. *The person with Alzheimer's disease: Pathways to understanding the experience*. Baltimore: Johns Hopkins University Press.

Hauerwas, S. 1986. *Suffering presence: Theological reflections on medicine, the mentally handicapped, and the church*. Notre Dame, IN: University of Notre Dame Press.

Hauerwas, S., and M. L. Budde. 2000. *The Ekklesia Project: A school for subversive friendships*. Ekklesia Project, Pamphlet #1. Available from www.ekklesiaproject.org.

Hauerwas, S., and Yordy, L. 2003. Captured in time: Friendship and aging. In S. Hauerwas, C. B. Stoneking., K. G. Meador, and D. Cloutier, eds., *Growing old in Christ*, 169–84. Grand Rapids, MI: William B. Eerdmans Publishing Co.

Hellebrandt, F. A. 1978. Comment—The senile dement in our midst: A look at the other side of the coin. *Gerontologist* 18:67–70.

Hellström, I., Nolan, M., and Lundh, U. 2005. "We do things together": A case study of "couplehood" in dementia. *Dementia* 4:7–22.

Hess, B. 1972. Friendship. In M. W. Riley, M. Johnson, and A. Foner, eds., *Aging and Society* 3:357–93. New York: Russell Sage Foundation.

Hirschberger, G., V. Florian, and M. Mikulincer. 2005. Fear and compassion: A terror management analysis of emotional reactions to disability. *Rehabilitation Psychology* 50:246–57.

Holstein, M. 2008. Fear, trembling, and hope: Alzheimer's and modern consciousness. *Gerontologist* 48:258–61.

Hughes, J. C., ed. 2006. Introduction: The heat of mild cognitive impairment. [Special issue]. *Philosophy, Psychiatry, and Psychology* 13(1).

Isaacowitz, D. M., H. A. Wadlinger, D. Goren, and H. R. Wilson. 2006. Selective preference in visual fixation away from negative images in old age? An eye-tracking study. *Psychology and Aging* 21:40–48.

James, W. 1890/1950. *The principles of psychology*. New York: Dover.

Kahn, R. L., and T. C. Antonucci. 1980. Convoys over the life course: Attachment, roles, and social support. In P. B. Baltes and O. G. Brim, eds., *Life span development and behavior* 3:253–86. New York: Academic Press.

Kastenbaum, R. 1993. Encrusted elders: Arizona and the political spirit of postmodern aging. In T. R. Cole, W. A. Achenbaum, P. L. Jakobi, and R. Kastenbaum, eds., *Voices and visions of aging: Toward a critical gerontology*, 160–83. New York: Springer Publishing Co.

Kastenbaum, R. 2004. *On our way: The final passage through life and death.* Berkeley: University of California Press.

Katsuno, T. 2005. Dementia from the inside: How people with early-stage dementia evaluate their quality of life. *Ageing and Society* 25:197–214.

Kegan, R. 1982. *The evolving self: Problem and process in human development.* Cambridge, MA: Harvard University Press.

Kenyon, G., P. Clark, and B. deVries, eds. 2001. *Narrative gerontology: Theory, research, and practice.* New York: Springer Publishing Co.

Kenyon, G. M., and W. L. Randall. 2001. Narrative gerontology: An overview. In Kenyon, Clark, and deVries, *Narrative gerontology,* 3–18.

Kessler, L. 2007. *Dancing with Rose: Finding life in the land of Alzheimer's.* New York: Viking.

Kimble, M. A., S. H. McFadden, J. W. Ellor, and J. J. Seeber, eds. 1995. *Aging, spirituality, and religion: A handbook.* Vol. 1. Minneapolis: Fortress Press.

Kimble, M. A., and S. H, McFadden, eds. 2003. *Aging, spirituality, and religion: A handbook.* Vol. 2. Minneapolis: Fortress Press.

Kitwood, T. 1997. *Dementia reconsidered: The person comes first.* Philadelphia: Open University Press.

Kleinman, A. 1988. *The illness narratives: Suffering, healing, and the human condition.* New York: Basic Books.

Knapp, J. L. 2003. *The graying of the flock: A new model for ministry.* Orange, CA: Leafwood Publishers.

Koenig, H. G., L. K. George, and I. C. Siegler. 1988. The use of religion and other emotion-regulating coping strategies among older adults. *Gerontologist* 28:303–10.

Kontos, P. 1998. Resisting institutionalization: Constructing old age and negotiating home. *Journal of Aging Studies* 12:167–84.

Krause, N. M. 2008. *Aging in the church: How social relationships affect health.* West Conshohocken, PA: Templeton Foundation Press.

Langdon, S. A., A. Eagle, and J. Warner. 2007. Masking sense of dementia in the social world: A qualitative study. *Social Science and Medicine* 64: 989–1000.

Lawton, M. P., and E. M. Brody. 1969. Assessment of older people: Self-maintaining and instrumental activities of daily living. *Gerontologist* 9:179–86.

Lazarus, R. S. 1991. *Emotion and adaptation.* New York: Oxford University Press.

Lazarus, R. S., and B. N. Lazarus. 2006. *Coping with aging.* New York: Oxford University Press.

Lewis, M., and J. M. Haviland-Jones, eds. 2000. *Handbook of emotions,* 2nd ed. New York: Guilford Press.

Lewis, T., F. Amini, and R. Lannon. 2000. *A general theory of love.* New York: Random House.

Lunsman, M. 2006. *College students' perceptions of old and young targets with health labels.* Master's thesis. University of Wisconsin, Oshkosh.

Luria, A. R. 1968/1987. *The mind of a mnemonist: A little book about a vast memory.* Cambridge, MA: Harvard University Press.

Lyman, K. A. 1998. Living with Alzheimer's disease: The creation of meaning among persons with dementia. *Journal of Clinical Ethics* 9:49–57.

MacDonald, G., and M. R. Leary. 2005. Why does social exclusion hurt? The relationship between social and physical pain. *Psychological Bulletin* 131:202–23.

Mace, N. L., and P. V. Rabins. 2006. *The 36-hour day: A family guide to caring for Alzheimer's disease, other dementias, and memory loss in later life.* 4th ed. Baltimore: Johns Hopkins University Press.

MacIntyre, A. 1999. *Dependent rational animals: Why human beings need the virtues.* Chicago: Open Court.

MacKinlay, E. 2001. *The spiritual dimension of ageing.* London: Jessica Kingsley Publishers.

MacKinlay, E. 2008a. Introduction: Ageing, disability, and spirituality. In MacKinlay, *Ageing, disability, and spirituality,* 11–21.

MacKinlay, E. 2008b. New and old challenges of ageing: Disabilities, spirituality and pastoral responses. In MacKinlay, *Ageing, disability, and spirituality,* 45–56.

MacKinlay, E., ed. 2008. *Ageing, disability, and spirituality: Addressing the challenge of disability in later life.* Philadelphia: Jessica Kingsley Publishers.

MacKinlay, E., and C. Trevitt. 2006. *Facilitating spiritual reminiscence for older people with dementia: A learning package.* Canberra: Centre for Ageing and Pastoral Studies.

Macmurray, J. 1957. *The self as agent.* London: Faber & Faber.

Macmurray, J. 1961. *Persons in relation.* London: Faber & Faber.

Marris, P. 2002. Holding onto meaning through the life cycle. In Weiss and Bass, *Challenges of the third age,* 13–28.

Martens, A., J. L. Goldenberg, and J. Greenberg. 2005. A terror management perspective on ageism. *Journal of Social Issues* 61:223–39.

Matthews, S. H. 1986. *Friendships through the life course: Oral biographies in old age.* Beverly Hills, CA: Sage Publications.

Matthews, S. H. 1996. Friendships in old age. In N. Vanzetti and S. Duck, eds., *A lifetime of relationships,* 406–30. Pacific Grove, CA: Brooks/Cole.

McCurdy, D. B. 1998. Personhood, spirituality, and hope in the care of human beings with dementia. *Journal of Clinical Ethics* 91:81–91.

McFadden, S. H. 2008. Mindfulness, vulnerability and love: Spiritual lessons from frail elders, earnest young pilgrims, and middle aged rockers. *Journal of Aging Studies* 22:132–39.

McFadden, S. H., and R. C. Atchley, eds. 2001. *Aging and the meaning of time: A multidisciplinary exploration.* New York: Springer Publishing Co.

McFadden, S. H., and A. D. Basting. 2010. Healthy aging persons and their brains: Promoting resilience through creative engagement. *Clinics in Geriatric Medicine* 26:149–61.

McFadden, S. H., M. Ingram, and C. Baldauf. 2000. Actions, feelings, and values: Foundations of meaning and personhood in dementia. *Journal of Religious Gerontology* 11(3/4):67–86.

McFadden, S. H., and J. Ramsey. 2010. Encountering the numinous: Relationality, the arts, and religion in later life. In T. R. Cole, R. E. Ray, and R. Kastenbaum, eds., *A guide to humanistic studies in aging: What does it mean to grow old?* 163–81. Baltimore: Johns Hopkins University Press.

McFadden, S. H., and J. Thibault. 2001. *Chronos* to *kairos*: Christian perspectives on time and aging. In McFadden and Atchley, *Aging and the meaning of time*, 229–50.

McKim, D. K., ed. 1997. *God never forgets: Faith, hope, and Alzheimer's disease*. Louisville, KY: Westminster John Knox Press.

McPherson, M., L. Smith-Lovin, and M. E. Brashears. 2006. Social isolation in America: Changes in core discussion networks over two decades. *American Sociological Review* 71:353–75.

Merchant, R. 2003. *Pioneering the third age: The church in an ageing population*. Waynesboro, GA: Paternoster Press.

Mitchell, A. J., and M. Shiri-Feshki. 2009. Rate of progression of mild cognitive impairment to dementia: Meta-analysis of 41 robust inception cohort studies. *Acta Psychiatrica Scandinavica* 119:252–65.

Modrego, P. J., N. Fayed, and M. A. Pina. 2005. Conversion from mild cognitive impairment to probable Alzheimer's disease predicted by brain magnetic resonance spectroscopy. *American Journal of Psychiatry* 162:667–75.

Moody, H. R. 1986. The meaning of life and the meaning of old age. In T. R. Cole and S. Gadow, eds., *What does it mean to grow old? Reflections from the humanities*, 11–40. Durham, NC: Duke University Press.

Moody, H. R. 2002. The changing meaning of aging. In Weiss and Bass, *Challenges of the third age*, 41–54.

Moremen, R. D. 2008. The downside of friendship: Sources of strain in older women's friendships. *Journal of Women and Aging* 20:169–87.

Morgan, R. 1996. *Remembering your story: A guide for spiritual autobiography*. Nashville, TN: Upper Room Press.

Morris, J. C. 2006. Mild cognitive impairment is early-stage Alzheimer disease: Time to revise diagnostic criteria. *Archives of Neurology* 63:115–16.

Morrow-Howell, N., J. Hinterlong, P. A. Rozario, and F. Tang. 2003. Effects of volunteering on the well-being of older adults. *Journal of Gerontology: Social Sciences* 58B:S137–45.

Newsom, C. A. 1996. The book of Job: Introduction, commentary, and reflections. In *The new interpreter's Bible: General articles and introduction, commentary, and reflections for each book of the Bible, including the apocryphal/deuterocanonical books in twelve volumes*, 4: 319–637. Nashville, TN: Abingdon Press.

Nouwen, H. 1988. *The road to Daybreak: A spiritual journey*. New York: Doubleday.

Nouwen, H. 1997. *Adam: God's beloved*. London: Darton, Longman & Todd.

Nowak, L., and J. E. Davis. 2007. A qualitative examination of the phenomenon of sundowning. *Journal of Nursing Scholarship* 39:256–58.

Nussbaum, J. F. 1994. Friendship in older adulthood. In M. L. Hummert, J. M. Wieman, and J. F. Nussbaum, eds., *Interpersonal communication in older adulthood: Interdisciplinary theory and research*, 209–25. Thousand Oaks, CA: Sage Publications.

Nussbaum, M. 2001. *Upheavals of thought: The intelligence of emotions*. New York: Cambridge University Press.

Öhman, A. 2000. Fear and anxiety: Evolutionary, cognitive, and clinical perspectives. In Lewis and Haviland-Jones, *Handbook of emotions*, 573–93.

Okun, M. A., and A. Schultz. 2003. Age and motives for volunteering: Testing hypotheses derived from socioemotional selectivity theory. *Psychology and Aging* 18:231–39.

Oman, D., C. E. Thoresen, and K. McMahon. 1999. Volunteerism and mortality among community-dwelling elderly. *Journal of Health Psychology* 4:301–16.

Pargament, K. I. 1997. *The psychology of religion and coping.* New York: Guilford Press.

Payne, B. P., and S. H. McFadden. 1994. From loneliness to solitude: Religious and spiritual journeys in late life. In L. E. Thomas and S. A. Eisenhandler, eds., *Aging and the religious dimension,* 13–27. Westport, CT: Auburn House.

Petersen, R. C. 2004. Mild cognitive impairment represents early-stage Alzheimer disease. *Journal of Internal Medicine* 256:183–94.

Plassman, B. L., K. M. Langa, G. G. Fisher, S. G. Heeringa, D. R. Weir, M. B. Ofstedal, et al. 2007. Prevalence of dementia in the United States: The aging, demographics, and memory study. *Neuroepidemiology* 29:125–32.

Plassman, B. L., K. M. Langa, G. G. Fisher, S. G. Heeringa, D. R. Weir, M. B. Ofstedal, et al. 2008. Prevalence of cognitive impairment without dementia in the United States. *Annals of Internal Medicine* 148:427–34.

Portet, F., P. J. Ousset, P. J. Visser, G. B. Frisoni, F. Nobili, P. Scheltens, et al. 2006. Mild cognitive impairment (MCI) in medical practice: A critical review of the concept and new diagnostic procedure. Report of the MCO Working Group of the European Consortium on Alzheimer's Disease. *Journal of Neurology, Neurosurgery, and Psychiatry* 7:714–18.

Post, S. G. 1995. *The moral challenge of Alzheimer disease.* Baltimore: Johns Hopkins University Press.

Powers, B. A. 1996. Relationships among older women living in a nursing home. *Journal of Women and Aging* 8:179–98.

Pratt, R., and H. Wilkinson. 2003. A psychosocial model of understanding the experience of receiving a diagnosis of dementia. *Dementia* 2: 181–99.

Purser, J., G. G. Fillenbaum, and R. B. Wallace. 2006. Memory complaint is not necessary for diagnosis of mild cognitive impairment and does not predict 10-year trajectories of functional disability, word recall, or Short Portable Mental Status Questionnaire limitations. *Journal of the American Geriatrics Society* 54:335–38.

Putnam, R. 1995. Bowling alone: American's declining social capital. *Journal of Democracy* 6:65–78.

Putnam, R. 2000. *Bowling alone: The collapse and revival of American community.* New York: Simon & Schuster.

Putnam, R., and D. Campbell. 2010. *American grace: How religion is reshaping our civic and political lives.* New York: Simon & Schuster.

Putnam, R., and L. M. Feldstein. 2003. *Better together: Restoring the American community.* New York: Simon & Schuster.

Rawlins, W. K. 1994. Being there and growing apart: Sustaining friendships during adulthood. In D. J. Canary and L. Stafford, eds., *Communication and relational maintenance.* San Diego: Academic Press.

Ray, R. 1996. A postmodern perspective on feminist gerontology. *Gerontologist* 36:674–80.

Reik, T. 1948. *Listening with the third ear: The inner experience of a psychoanalyst.* New York: Farrar, Strauss.

Reinders, H. S. 2008. *Receiving the gift of friendship: Profound disability, theological anthropology, and ethics.* Ann Arbor, MI: Eerdmans.

Reisberg, B., S. H. Ferris, M. J. DeLeon, and T. Crook. 1982. The Global Deterioration Scale for assessment of primary degenerative dementia. *American Journal of Psychiatry* 139:1136–39.

Reynolds, T. 2008. *Vulnerable communion: A theology of disability and hospitality.* Grand Rapids, MI: Brazos Press.

Rieff, P. 1966. *The triumph of the therapeutic: Uses of faith after Freud.* New York: Harper & Row.

Roberto, K. A. 1996. Friendships between older women: Interactions and reactions. In K. A. Roberto, ed., *Relationships between women in later life,* 55–73. New York: Harrington Park Press.

Robertson, A. 1990. The politics of Alzheimer's disease: A case study in apocalyptic demography. *International Journal of Health Services* 20:429–42.

Rook, K. S. 1989. Strains in older adults' friendships. In R. G. Adams and R. Blieszner, eds., *Older adult friendship: Structure and process,* 166–94. Newbury Park, CA: Sage Publications.

Rook, K. S., and D. H. Sorkin. 2003. Fostering social ties through a volunteer role: Implications for older-adults' psychological health. *International Journal of Aging and Human Development* 57:313–37.

Rosen, H. J., K. Pace-Savitsky, R. J. Perry, J. H. Kramer, B. L. Miller, and R. W. Levenson. 2004. Recognition of emotion in the frontal and temporal variants of frontotemporal dementia. *Dementia and Geriatric Cognitive Disorders* 17:277–81.

Rosow, I. 1967. *Social integration of the aged.* New York: Free Press.

Royce, J. R. 1973. The present situation in theoretical psychology. In B. B. Wolman, ed., *Handbook of general psychology,* 8–21. Englewood Cliffs, NJ: Prentice Hall.

Rozin, P., J. Haidt, and C. R. McCauley. 2000. Disgust. In Lewis and Haviland-Jones, *Handbook of emotions,* 637–53.

Rubinstein, R. L. 2002. The third age. In Weiss and Bass, *Challenges of the third age,* 29–40.

Ryan, E. B., L. S. Martin, and A. Beaman. 2005. Communication strategies to promote spiritual well-being among people with dementia. *Journal of Pastoral Care and Counseling* 59:43–55.

Sabat, S. R. 2001. *The experience of Alzheimer's disease: Life through a tangled veil.* Malden, MA: Blackwell Publishers.

Scholl, J. M., and S. R. Sabat. 2008. Stereotypes, stereotype threat and ageing: Implications for the understanding and treatment of people with Alzheimer's disease. *Ageing and Society* 28:103–30.

Seman, D. 2002. Meaningful communication throughout the journey: Clinical observations. In Harris, *The person with Alzheimer's disease,* 134–49.

Shamy, E. 2003. *A guide to the spiritual dimension of care for people with Alzheimer's disease and related dementia: More than body, brain, and breath.* New York: Jessica Kingsley Publishers.

Shmotkin, D., T. Blumstein, and B. Modan. 2003. Beyond keeping active: Concomitants of being a volunteer in old-old age. *Psychology and Aging* 18:602–7.

Shuman, J. J. 2009. God does not wear a white coat—but God does heal. In D. B. Laytham, ed., *God does not . . . entertain, play "matchmaker," hurry, demand blood, cure every illness*, 21–38. Grand Rapids, MI: Brazos Press.

Sifton, C. B. 2004. *Navigating the Alzheimer's journey: A compass for caregiving*. Baltimore: Health Professions Press.

Simard, J., and L. Volicer. 2010. Effects of Namaste Care on residents who do not benefit from usual activities. *American Journal of Alzheimer's Disease and Other Dementias* 25: 46–50.

Slater, P. 1976. *The pursuit of loneliness: American culture at the breaking point*. Boston: Beacon Press.

Slife, B. D. 2004. Taking practice seriously: Toward a relational ontology. *Journal of Theoretical and Philosophical Psychology* 24:157–78.

Smith, G., and B. K. Rush. 2006. Normal aging and mild cognitive impairment. In Attix and Welsh-Bohmer, *Geriatric neuropsychology*, 27–55.

Snyder, L. 2009. *Speaking our minds: What it's like to have Alzheimer's*. Rev. ed. Baltimore: Health Professions Press.

Snowden, D. 2001. *Aging with grace: What the nun study teaches us about leading longer, healthier, and more meaningful lives*. New York: Bantam Books.

Solomon, S., J. Greenberg, and T. Pyszczynski. 2004. The cultural animal: Twenty years of terror management theory and research. In Greenberg, Koole, and Pyszczynski, *Handbook of experimental existential psychology*, 13–34.

Sontag, S. 1977. *Illness as metaphor*. New York: Ferrar, Straus & Giroux.

Stansell, J. 2002. Volunteerism: Contributions by persons with Alzheimer's disease. In Harris, *The person with Alzheimer's disease*, 211–27.

Stein, R. 2008. One-third of seniors have mental decline: Large number surprises researchers. *Washington Post*, March 18, A3.

Swinton, J. 2000. *Resurrecting the person: Friendship and the care of people with mental health problems*. Nashville, TN: Abingdon Press.

Swinton, J., ed. 2004. Critical reflections on Stanley Hauerwas' theology of disability: Disabling society, enabling theology [Special issue]. *Journal of Religion, Disability and Health* 8(3/4).

Swinton, J. 2007. Forgetting whose we are: Theological reflections on personhood, faith and dementia. *Journal of Religion, Disability, and Health* 11:37–63.

Swinton, J. 2008. The body of Christ has Down syndrome: Theological reflections on vulnerability, disability, and graceful communities. University of Aberdeen, Centre for Spirituality, Health, and Disability Website: www.abdn.ac.uk/cshad/TheBodyof ChristHasDownSyndrome.htm

Swinton, J., and B. Brock, eds. 2007. *Theology, disability and the new genetics*. London: T & T Clark.

Swinton, J., and E. McIntosh. 2000. Persons in relation: The care of persons with learning disabilities. *Theology Today* 57:175–84.

Taylor, R. 2007. *Alzheimer's from the inside out*. Baltimore: Health Professions Press.

Taylor, R. J., L. M. Chatters, and J. S. Jackson. 2007. Religious and spiritual involvement among older African Americans, Caribbean Blacks, and non-Hispanic Whites: Findings from the National Survey of American Life. *Journal of Gerontology: Social Sciences* 62B:S238–50.

Tillich, P. 1957. *Dynamics of faith*. New York: Harper & Row.

Traphagen, J. W. 2000. *Taming oblivion: Aging bodies and the fear of senility in Japan*. Albany, NY: State University of New York Press.

Trevitt, C., and E. MacKinlay. 2006. "I am just an ordinary person . . .": Spiritual reminiscence in older people with memory loss. *Journal of Religion, Spirituality, and Aging* 18:79–91.

Vanier, J. 1998. *Becoming human*. Mahwah, NJ: Paulist Press.

Vernooij-Dassen, M., E. Derksen, P. Scheltens, and E. Moniz-Cook. 2006. Receiving a diagnosis of dementia: The experience over time. *Dementia* 5:397–410.

Volf, M. 1996. *Exclusion and Embrace: A theological exploration of identity, otherness, and reconciliation*. Nashville, TN: Abingdon Press.

Weiss, R. S., and S. A. Bass. 2002. *Challenges of the third age: Meaning and purpose in later life*. New York: Oxford University Press.

Welsh-Bohmer, K. A., and L. H. Warren. 2006. Neurodegenerative dementias. In Attix and Welsh-Bohmer, *Geriatric neuropsychology*, 56–88.

Whitehouse, P. J. 2006. Demystifying the mystery of Alzheimer's as late, no longer mild cognitive impairment. *Philosophy, Psychiatry, and Psychology* 13:87–88.

Whitehouse, P. J., and D. George. 2008. *The myth of Alzheimer's: What you aren't being told about today's most dreaded diagnosis*. New York: St. Martin's Press.

Whitehouse, P. J., K. Maurer, and J. F. Ballenger, eds. 2000. *Concepts of Alzheimer disease: Biological, clinical, and cultural perspectives*. Baltimore: Johns Hopkins University Press.

Whitehouse, P. J., and H. R. Moody. 2006. Mild cognitive impairment: A "hardening of the categories"? *Dementia* 5:11–25.

Wilz, G., and M. Fink-Heitz. 2008. Assisted vacations for men with dementia and their caregiving spouses: Evaluation of health-related effects. *Gerontologist* 48:115–20.

Wolfe, T. 1976. The "me" decade and the third great awakening. *New York Magazine*, August 23.

Zakaria, F. 1996. The ABCs of communitarianism: A devil's dictionary. www.slate.com/id/2380/.

Zandi, R., M. Cooper, and L. Garrison. 1992. Facial recognition: A cognitive study of elderly dementia patients and normal older adults. *International Psychogeriatrics* 4:215–21.

Zhong, C.-B., and G. J. Leonardelli. 2008. Cold and lonely: Does social exclusion literally feel cold? *Psychological Science* 19:838–42.

Zinnbauer, B. J., K. I. Pargament, B. Cole, M. S. Rye, E. M. Butter, T. G. Belavich, et al. 1997. Religion and spirituality: Unfuzzying the fuzzy. *Journal for the Scientific Study of Religion* 36:549–64.

Susan H. McFadden, Ph.D., is Professor Emerita of Psychology at the University of Wisconsin Oshkosh, where she continues to conduct research and teach part-time. She is also the research consultant for the Fox Valley Memory Project (www.foxval leymemoryproject.org), which is creating an integrative, multi-faceted model of a dementia-friendly community in northeast Wisconsin. She is a fellow of Division 36 (Society for the Psychology of Religion and Spirituality) of the American Psychological Association, which honored her in 2013 with the William C. Bier Award for contributions to the field of psychology, religion, and spirituality. She co-edited the two volumes of *Aging, Spirituality, and Religion: A Handbook.* Other co-edited books include *New Directions in the Study of Late Life Religiousness and Spirituality, Aging and the Meaning of Time,* and *Handbook of Emotion, Adult Development, and Aging.* She has published more than thirty journal articles and book chapters on the psychology of aging, especially as related to older adults' religiousness, spirituality, and creativity.

John T. McFadden, M.Div., is an ordained minister of the United Church of Christ who served in parish ministry for thirty-four years, including twenty-three years as senior pastor of First Congregational United Church of Christ in Appleton, Wisconsin. He currently serves as Memory Care Chaplain at the Appleton Health Care Center and as an advocate for community-based programs for innovative dementia care promoted by the Fox Valley Memory Project. He has written two books. *Bear Suit Follies: The Songs, Stories, and Letters of Antonia* tells the story of Antonia Stampfel, a long-time friend. Once active in the 1960s and 1970s rock and roll music scene in New York City, she now lives in an assisted-living residence in Florida, where she still writes songs despite a stroke and numerous other afflictions of age. His other book, *The Open Door: A History of First Congregational Church, 1850–2000,* won the Wisconsin Historical Society's award of merit in 2000. John has also written several monographs and book chapters.